Madness Reimagined

Envisioning a Better System of Mental Health in America

Leonard A. Steverson
Flagler College; USA

Cognitive Science and Psychology
VERNON PRESS

www.vernonpress.com

In the Americas:
Vernon Press
1000 N West Street,
Suite 1200, Wilmington,
Delaware 19801
United States

In the rest of the world:
Vernon Press
C/Sancti Espiritu 17,
Malaga, 29006
Spain

Cognitive Science and Psychology

Library of Congress Control Number: 2018951086

ISBN: 978-1-62273-328-6

Cover design by Vernon Press using elements designed by Freepik.

Table of Contents

PREFACE

Madness Reimagined is an analysis of the current mental health system in America. It begins with the history of the treatment of people with mental distress, as the past can function as a beacon to guide us into areas of new possibilities while avoiding the areas that proved to be hazardous in earlier times. The book acts as a guide to help navigate the current field regarding those behaviors and thought processes determined by our society to be mental disorders; to understand mental health classification and the Diagnostic and Statistical Manual of Mental Disorders; to recognize the various "psy-professionals" that provide mental health treatment; and to become acquainted with the major psychotherapy treatment models currently in use. It utilizes a sociological analysis to provide theoretical and conceptual underpinnings of mental health and illness and proposes a systems perspective to examine the component parts of the mental health system, as well as its relationship to other systems with which it engages.

The book also addresses the issue of advocacy for people who receive mental health services as well as for the services themselves. It attempts to create dialogues that will promote the reimagining process as it is felt that conversations that start by asking questions rather than presuming answers create more room for real examination, contemplation, and deliberation. The social constructionist approach used in the work offers a challenge to our understandings of mental health and mental illness and examines the role of cultural as well as natural realities. In this vein, the concept of therapeutic substructure—the underlying social aspects of the system—is introduced to assist in probing the cultural foundations of mental illness.

The information contained in these pages is meant to be jargon-free and accessible to a variety of publics, including mental health consumers and their families, advocates, mental health practitioners, students and trainees, as well as academics. In this way, it seeks to adopt features of public sociology by getting information into communities where community members can reimagine a better system and to put this reimagining into practice.

ACKNOWLEDGEMENTS

I would like to acknowledge the influences and support systems involved in this project. I am grateful for the people involved in my clinical training received quite a few years ago. I especially owe a debt of gratitude to my late professor, advisor, and dear friend John H. Curtis, a major influence on my understanding of mental health and mental illness.

I also wish to thank the staff at Flagler College's Proctor Library who put up with my consistent pestering for resources and did so with courteous accommodation. I also am appreciative to Meghan Durrance for assistance in the preparation of the manuscript and Amelia Clancy for her work on researching the resources in the final chapter; their contributions allowed me to finish the work while maintaining my own mental well-being.

And, as always, I wish to acknowledge the love and support of my soul mate, Betty, and our children and grandchildren who continue to be my inspiration. It is to them I dedicate this book.

Chapter 1

INTRODUCTION

"...the sociological imagination... is the capacity to shift from one perspective to another—from the political to the psychological; from examination of a single family to comparative assessments of the national budgets of the world..."

(C. Wright Mills, 1959 p. 7)

PURPOSE OF THE BOOK

The purpose of this book is to explore the system of mental health as it operates in the United States, to shed some light on the services provided in the mental health system, and to provide education about advocacy for people with mental illness. The work seeks to provide information on this important topic to the public in the hope that the knowledge will help people—people experiencing mental health problems, their families, early career mental health professionals, and the public generally—understand the nuances of the field of mental health. Most people understand the basics of mental health, and many suffer from what could be considered a mental disorder; certainly, everyone knows someone who is directly affected. But what is lesser known is how the *system* works and the ways in which it can be made better for millions of Americans. A better understanding of the system, with its history, component parts, and many nuances, should be a requirement for all new therapists and therapy students—this is something the author wishes he had experienced prior to entering the field.

The first word in the book's title is *madness*. This is because the term was common in an earlier time to describe mental illness; it carries with it a long history that, when we reflect on it, provides a valuable framework in which to understand our current treatment of mental illness. It is a term that reflects the pain and misery that has been inflicted upon people since antiquity, a pain that permeates into families, communities, and society in general. The idea was that people who lost their senses or rationality were *mad* and unable to function appropriately. Mental illness was, in fact, considered deviant behavior, even though it was understood that sufferers were often not in control of their faculties. Deviance, after all, refers to behavior that goes against ("deviates" from) social norms. Referring to health in a general sense, one social scientist (Turney-High, 1968) noted in a textbook years ago, "...those in poor health are among the not needed, not wanted, but here..." (p. 562); this statement reflects the misery of many with a mental disability.

In the twentieth century, the term psychosis was used to define what was formerly called madness, lunacy, and insanity (Torrey & Miller, 2001). Torrey and Miller's (2001) definition of insanity (and by extension, madness), includes schizophrenia, schizoaffective disorders, delusional disorder, and depressive disorder with psychotic features; this categorization excludes non-psychotic disorders. This concept of madness is too limited and excludes many disorders that have throughout history had this designation. For example, actions of a person behaving erratically under the influence of drugs, or socio-pathologically harming others have been considered acts of madness. Likewise, more internalized behaviors such as engaging in ritualistic behaviors that cause disfigurement to the body, or excessive fears that are irrational have also been considered madness. And, of course, these behaviors have a home in the Diagnostic and Statistical Manual of Mental Disorders (or DSM, the official diagnostic guide for mental illness) in the form of substance use disorder, antisocial personality disorder, obsessive-compulsive disorder, and specific phobia. The point here is not to label these behaviors as madness but to point out that historically many behaviors once considered madness, and currently considered mental illness, are pervasive. And many of us who don't have an official clinical diagnosis could easily be given such a label. The cat in Alice's Adventures in Wonderland perhaps had it right, "we're all mad here".

Madness is often understood to include conditions that are "severe" such as psychosis or other extreme manifestations of mental problems. However, if we take a seemingly minor, benign condition such as phobia, and then observe the potential severe phobic reactions to things such as insects, snakes, germs, or other stimuli, we realize it is not so minor at all. Another example is an obsessive-compulsive disorder, which is characterized by obsessive thoughts that are followed by ritualistic, repetitive behavior—while this might seem as simply odd and quirky to outsiders, it can be exasperating to sufferers. To assume that these experiences do not have "maddening" effects to the sufferers would be wrong and disrespect their plight. Therefore, most mental conditions produce varying degrees of individual distress and dysfunction, and one cannot assume that some perceived inconsequential problems do not have the ability to be disabling. Therefore, this book will examine many types of mental disorder in its analysis of "madness".

It is commonly accepted that we have made great advancements as a society in treating what was once called madness. Improvements in treatment modalities that are inspired by scientific research, medical treatments, and a progressive focus on diagnosis, have made the mental health field much different than it was in the past. In chapter two, we will see just how far the field has advanced. The advances we have experienced reflect a level of optimism that these ailments could be cured—as we will see, often these imaginings took the form of some very unscientific (and even unscrupulous) methods; however, they have moved us in the direction of a better understanding of the causes and potential treatment of mental illness.

The word *reimagined* is used in this book to reflect the idea that although progress has been made, greater visions are needed to advance us further, especially considering the potential barriers that threaten the care and treatment of the mentally ill. In addition, those who suffer from mental illness experience anguish from the stigma of their condition, as many in society still cast an unfavorable eye on the disorders and the people who must deal with it on a day-to-day basis. It's as if the disorders associated with it aren't bad enough—the response from the public simply worsens the situation. Although physical illness bears some social stigma, it often pales in comparison to that generated by mental illness. "Madness" must be reimagined and it is through educating the public that this reimagining will begin.

The term *envision* infers a process that seeks to promote a positive vision of change. Through a concerted effort, which includes policy changes and advocacy, this positive change can be realized. Better living conditions for those with mental illness is not just a benefit to those individuals, but society in general. To envision a better society requires a focus on social justice, which has deep philosophical roots and includes not only the idea that a society should have a stable and consistent set of rules and moral codes, but the rules and codes should also be enacted in a way as to improve equal treatment of its citizens. This process requires that agreements to assist those in need be kept (Frankena, 1962). This idea suggests there is a social contract that exists between members of society and their social institutions in which citizens must become involved to ensure equal and just treatment of all people. Advocacy and social justice in the field of mental health will be examined in more detail in chapter seven.

The subtitle reveals an important emphasis of this work; that of mental health as a *system.* A systems approach requires us to conceptualize social approaches to mental health as operating in a structure with interconnected component parts that work in conjunction with other systems, such as the health system generally, the criminal justice system, social service systems, and others. The effectiveness of the mental health system is closely aligned with the effectiveness of these other systems. This idea of a systems approach will be discussed in more detail in chapter six.

UNDERSTANDING MENTAL ILLNESS AND SUBSTANCE USE DISORDER

Mental Illness

What we understand as mental illness is a topic that intrigues many people. It is the subject of movies, books, art, music, and many news stories that focus on people with mental problems. It is certainly not uncommon to encounter people with severe and chronic mental illness; in fact, most of us encounter people with less severe forms daily—we are often just not aware of it. It affects people of all ages, both genders, people of all racial and ethnic groups and nationalities, indeed, people of every conceivable type.

It is illuminating to look at some facts and figures regarding mental illness in America. The National Institute of Mental Health (NIMH), the governmental agency providing information that assists in "understanding and treating mental illness" (NIMH, n.d., para. 1), has data for differentiating "any mental illness" and "severe mental illness". Any mental illness (AMI) refers to an illness (mental, behavioral, or emotional) that is currently diagnosable (or diagnosed with the past year), and experience no, mild, or severe impairment. Over 43 million Americans (about 18% of all citizens) aged 18 or over are experiencing disorders in the AMI illness category. A severe mental illness (SMI) is one in which people are currently diagnosable (or diagnosed within the past year) and experience serious and enduring impairments that interfere with major life activities. Nearly 10 million people (4%) of this age group are experiencing disorders in the severe (SMI) category. Regarding young people in the 13- to 18-year age group, over 46% have AMI and 21% have an SMI; it is certainly disturbing to note that 1 in 5 children have a debilitating mental condition (NIMH, n.d.). Therefore, as these data show, many people experience mental illness in some form during their lives. And ALL of us are affected by it in some way.

To fully understand an institution such as the health care system, it must be analyzed from the historical process that produced it (Berger & Luckmann, 1966). The term "produced" is important here as it reflects the idea that various parts of society, including our conceptions of mental health and mental illness, are products of our cultural history rather than a distinct, naturally occurring process. Humans decided what constituted mental health and mental illness (and continue to construct them) as well as the system that encompassed these constructions—the mental health system. Therefore, this book looks at the mental health system from this lens—as a system created by people based on how we construct meaning informed by a long and complex history that must be understood from social and contextual factors. This approach, called social constructionism, is one of the theoretical underpinnings of the book.

It is suggested here that madness is a social construction. What this means is that we as humans create words and concepts to describe some common understandings of things, to make sense of the world and to communicate with others. Madness is such a construction. What does it mean to be "mad"? Moving from its most common usage as a state of being angry; an alternative meaning, also clearly understood by most in the English-speaking world, is a state of mental disturbance or mental illness. Since we are unable to find a definition of the term madness in the scientific literature, we will refer to Merriam-Webster's Dictionary (2018), which defines this form of madness in a variety of ways with concepts for which we have some degree of familiarity: "foolishness", "dangerousness", "extreme folly", "ecstasy", "enthusiasm", "rage", "frenzied behavior", and of course, "mental illness". The American Heritage Dictionary (2000) adds that madness means "deranged", a term that refers to a condition that disturbs the order, arrangement, and functioning of an individual—the word "order" is instructive as it implies there is a natural order that has been disturbed in people who are mad. And this assumes that madness, or mental illness, is considered a deviant condition which, as we will soon see, was a major focus of labeling theorists.

Scull (2015) rejects the idea of madness as a social construction, stating it reduces mental illness to a state of consciousness devoid of reality. This, however, seems to miss the point. It is not that people do not really experience the traumatic effects of mental illness—people do actually struggle with hallucinations and delusions, tormenting obsessions, withdrawal symptoms related to addiction and many other symptoms as well as the accompanying stigma from both the sufferer and those who observe them. The idea of social constructionism means we observe and categorize social phenomena in a way that is one option among many others.

Social constructionism forces us to understand why we develop understandings of and hence categorize things as we do. If we look at, for example, how the DSM is organized, much thought went into what determines its classification as a mental disorder, what constitutes its features, how the disorders are grouped together, etc. Likewise, the way in which this book was organized—the chapters that were selected, the arrangement of the chapters, the sources used, the theoretical perspective adopted, the decision to adopt a public sociology approach, and many others were but of a few choices of innumerable possibilities. But we must look at all the other ways things could have been organized, to formulate a complete picture of what is considered mental illness.

We realize that some things that were considered mental disorders at one time, such as hysteria and neurasthenia, are no longer considered human conditions at all. Some conditions maintained their designation as mental disorders, but the names were changed, such as melancholia, manic depressive disorder, and dipsomania (now depression, bipolar disorder, and substance use disorder, respectively). And the fact that some identity issues such as homosexuality were once considered mental disorders, and now are not, makes it difficult to see mental disorders as naturally occurring conditions. Society has designated some conditions as mental disorders among a choice of many others. It is important to understand why this is so.

We must keep in mind the concept of the Thomas Theorem developed by W.I. Thomas (Thomas & Thomas, 1928) which states that even though aspects of life might not have a distinct reality (they are not real), the consequences of our beliefs about them are real. For example, when homosexuality was considered a mental disorder, it had distinct and broad consequences for gay people who were forced to remain "in the closet" and were blocked from positive aspects of life, including marriage.

Substance Use Disorders

This book is an analysis of the mental health system and includes the related issues of substance use disorders and addiction. To express the prevalence of substance abuse disorders and addiction, some statistics are in order. According to the Substance Abuse and Mental Health Services Administration (SAMHSA), a governmental agency that oversees the nation's substance abuse and mental health administration, 2015 data show that over 27 million people age 12 and older (1 in 10 Americans) took illegal drugs (hallucinogens, inhalants, methamphetamine) or misused legal drugs (such as prescribed medications) and nearly 21 million of the same age group has a substance use disorder (SUD) (SAMHSA, 2015).

Over 8 million people (or about 1 in 12) with SUDs that have co-occurring mental health disorders (AMI) and 48% are receiving some form of SUD treatment. Over 2 million adults have severe mental illness and almost 63% of this group are receiving SUD treatment. Among adolescents with a dual diagnosis of mental disorder and substance use disorder, 350,000 adolescents (1.4%), over 64% are receiving SUD treatment (Bose, Hedden, Lapari, & Park-Lee, 2016). As these statistics reveal, the issues of substance abuse and addiction are a serious issue in society. Over the last few years, it has been opiate addiction that has gained the attention of lawmakers nationwide as an epidemic concern, but the use of methamphetamine is also currently a major focus of drug policy (Vestal, 2017).

Developmental Disorders

This work excludes the issue of developmental disorders for several reasons. While mental illness, substance use disorders and developmental disorders are all considered part of the mental health care system, the issue of "madness" as addressed in this work implies a mental disturbance that causes erratic thoughts and/or behaviors that profoundly affects a person's life—mental illness and substance addiction (and the related issue of behavioral addictions which will be discussed soon) often lead to chaotic situations that are considered mental disturbances. And while both all three categories are included in the all-important Diagnostic Statistical Manual of Mental Disorders (DSM), developmental disabilities (identified as neurodevelopmental disorders which include intellectual disability, autism spectrum disorder, and attention-deficit/hyperactivity disorder, among others) occur early in a person's development and persist throughout that person's lifetime with somewhat limited benefits of external intervention, unlike mental illness and addiction, which occurs somewhere along a person's lifespan and whose positive treatment outcomes depend on external interventions. In other words, it is a cultural assumption that people "go mad" and that is not normally a consideration with developmental disorders.

Certainly, mental illness, substance use disorders and developmental disorders all receive stigmatic reactions from society (along with prejudice and discrimination) but the reactions are different as developmental disabilities do not tend to evoke opprobrious feelings as do mental disorders or substance abuse. In addition, the issue of recovery, for decades a major goal in substance abuse and now an evolving focus in mental health (Watson, 2012); recovery is not a treatment goal for developmental disorders. The related goal of relapse prevention is likewise not a treatment goal with the developmentally disabled, unless there is a co-occurring mental disorder or substance abuse condition. This is certainly not to say psychotherapy is not valuable to those with developmental disorders, but recovery and relapse prevention are not intended outcomes with this population not experiencing coexisting conditions.

SOCIOLOGY AND MENTAL HEALTH

Normally when issues concerning mental illness are explored, this analysis takes place within the framework of psychiatry, psychology, or biology. The biological sciences, including genetics, neuroscience, and pharmacology are currently prominent in understandings and treatment of mental (as well as physical) illness as these fields are experiencing several advancements, as well as increased media attention. In addition, they are often supported by medical doctors and professional medical associations, who have powerful voices in the mental health fields. Also, information derived from these fields is peremptorily accepted by many sufferers of mental illness, the public generally, and politicians, as they offer an easy explanation for mental problems by suggesting they are the result of biological effects in individuals rather than the complex of problems in society, thereby removing the responsibility of treatment from the patient to society. While the biologically-based disciplines do in some instances account for the role of social factors, their primary focus is obviously on the biological and constitutional features of illness (Busfield, 2000).

Therefore, in many ways, mental health would seem to be the providence of these biologically-focused disciplines. The social sciences, however, account for the environmental (social and cultural) aspects of humans and human behavior which is often lacking in the biological disciplines. Sociology is a social science discipline that seeks to understand how thoughts and behavior are influenced by social factors and how society, in turn, reacts to our behaviors. Sociology also addresses norms and reactions to violations of those norms; since mental illness is based on the recognition of a violation of norms, it has probably been around since the beginning of humanity. Daniel H. Tuke, British physician and specialist in mental health, explained that due to civilization's evolving complexity and the growing demands in people's lives, mental illness is increasing (Deutsch, 1949); the interesting thing is that this proclamation was made in 1892! The late twentieth century certainly had its hardships, but it is interesting to examine the new demands that we face as we settle into the 21st century.

Sociology steps back and looks at the bigger picture of social phenomena. This work, therefore, seeks to observe the system of mental health care in America. It looks at how mental health disorders are classified, how people with these disorders are affected, how the system has changed over time, and how society reacts to mental illness. Sociology observes social phenomena and social institutions with an eye on the effects of race, gender, class, ethnicity, sexual identity, and other prominent characteristics. One of sociology's greatest investigations has been around stigma, which refers to a visible sign that someone is different or possesses characteristics that are determined to be undesirable—stigma is something that has consistently plagued people with mental illness throughout history and it will be addressed in depth in this work.

Sociology has many branches, or subfields, including the sociology of race and ethnicity, sex and gender, deviance, stratification, and the sociology of institutions (the family, government, economy, religion, education), among many others. The sociology of mental health is a relatively new subfield of sociology and focuses on how society and social interactions are created and reinforced through norms (general expectations for people in society)—mental illness in its different forms is a violation of the norms. The mind is not separate from society. People follow the dictates of society and those who violate social norms must experience social sanctions.

An even newer branch is called public sociology and this subfield seeks to educate the public about social issues and institutions (in this case the mental health system) by providing information from a sociological perspective that is based on sociological research, theorizing, and things learned from the application of interventions that seek to improve these issues and institutions. Too often scholarly information is shared within the halls of academia, but it fails to find its way to the communities, groups, and local organizations that need this information to alleviate the social problems for which they were created. Public sociology seeks to remedy this by disseminating information to people and groups who need it; it is in this vein the book seeks to extend this knowledge on mental health and the mental health system to the public. It is the hope that this knowledge transfer will result in the reimagining of the current mental health system and the betterment of people's lives.

It would be useful now to review some of the commonly used definitions of the terms related to mental health and mental disorder. Most of these terms are probably familiar, however, they are often confused, used incorrectly or inappropriately, and used interchangeably (even if they are not the same thing). Therefore, this section should provide some clarity about terms in a system that can be mystifying and provide an introduction to the upcoming chapters.

MENTAL HEALTH AND MENTAL ILLNESS

We will start with the terms mental health and mental illness. *Mental health*, according to the World Health Organization (WHO), is more than the absence of diagnosable mental conditions—it is a requirement for the maintenance of the overall health of people and can be attributed to a host of socioeconomic and environmental conditions as well as biological factors (WHO, 2016). It is defined more specifically as "a state of well-being in which an individual realizes his or her own abilities, can cope with the normal stresses of life, can work productively and is able to make a contribution to his or her community" whereas poor mental health is "associated with rapid social change, stressful work conditions, physical ill-health and human rights violations" (WHO, 2016). Other terms, as we shall see, have been used throughout history to describe mental health in terms of sanity and mental hygiene. More recently, the term "behavioral health" has come into use, and though some people make some distinctions between this term and mental health (through the inclusion of substance use disorders as well), it is closely aligned to the more common term and, like mental health, is often used to differentiate itself from physical health. Despite some advantages to the term behavioral health, the more conventional term mental health will be used in this work.

The National Institute of Mental Health (NIMH) defines *mental illness* as "a mental, behavioral, or emotional disorder…of sufficient duration to meet diagnostic criteria…" (now of the DSM-5) (NIMH, n.d.) which refers to an individual's inability to effectively deal with the daily encounters in life. It should be obvious the terms mental health and mental illness are analogized with physical health. For a long time, the field of mental health was perceived to be an extension of physical health and one that could use the medical model to treat (and "cure") these ailments. There are many slang words that are informally used for mental illness that are derogatory and will not be mentioned in this work (except in their historical context) because these words are deeply insulting and demeaning. It is well known that mental illness often carries more stigma than physical health and this subject will be addressed later in the book.

It should also be noted that there are different types and levels of severity in mental illness. Although we use the term to mean different things, the fact that we often lump them together into one type is unfortunate. Mental health diagnoses are on a spectrum that run from severe mental problems such as schizophrenia and bipolar disorder to mild phobias or relationship problems. And within each of these classifications there are varying levels of severity of symptoms. A simple and useful distinction differentiates "acute" mental illness which is episodic and often involves reactions to stressful conditions, and "chronic" disorders that are severe and enduring (Scheid, 2004). One last note—the terms mental illness and mental disorder will be used throughout the text as this is current nomenclature, however, the use of these terms will be evaluated in chapter 8.

Psychopathology

Psychopathology is a term with clinical implications. The medical term "pathology" refers to the study of diseases and abnormalities while the prefix "psych" has mental or psychological connotations. Again, we can see the connection of mental health and mental illness to that of the physical, and how the use of the medical model is reflected in mental health treatment. With historical analysis, we can see the progression of understandings of mental illness as having a supernatural basis to the current medical approach.

Addictive Disorder

An *addictive disorder* refers to a disturbance of compulsive craving, either to a substance or a behavior. Traditionally, addictive disorders (called substance or chemical addictions) referred to those produced by the ingestion of a chemical agent such as alcohol, cocaine, heroin (among many others), which then produces an intoxicating effect on the brain, which can lead to addiction (also called habituation), a compulsive desire to use the drug again. Recently, however, activities such as gambling, sexual activity, have been posited to cause addictive responses (these are referred to as behavioral or process addictions). Substance and behavioral addictions can both result in significant disturbances for addicted people, as well as those of the people in their lives.

Mental Health Institutions

Mental health institutions normally refer to mental health hospitals and are places where persons with mental health issues are engaged in psychotherapy and other forms of treatment to alleviate the problems they are experiencing. Normally hospitalization is sought by people with more serious disorders. Mental health hospitals, with names of the past that might sound foreign to us now such as asylums, mad houses, insane hospitals, and lunatic hospitals, have a very long history in and will be examined soon. In addition, there are hospitals for those who have a specialty focus in working with people with addiction problems. Broader interpretations of institutions would include community-based clinics which offer a plethora of outpatient programs, covered later in this book.

Mental Health Diagnosis

Mental health diagnosis refers to the classification and labeling of the specific problem a client is experiencing. The process of diagnosis attempts to find common attributes of a certain condition and lump them together into a discernable category which allows practitioners to address the condition therapeutically. The term comorbidity refers to the presence of more than one disorder; this is not uncommon, however, and should not be understood as a rare occurrence. Another term is dual diagnosis, which refers to the co-occurrence of both a psychological disorder and a substance use disorder. Additionally, the term nosology which is also used in this book refers to how the medical system classifies disorders.

The primary instrument used in arriving at mental health diagnoses is the Diagnostic and Statistical Manual of Mental Disorders (which has produced several editions over the years), often shorted to the "DSM", and the current iteration is the DSM-5. This comprehensive manual provides diagnostic information about every condition that has been deemed to be a mental disorder and has experienced several revisions. Diagnosis and the DSM, including its evolution, will be discussed in more detail, along with the disorders and diagnosticians/practitioners in chapter three.

Psychotherapy

The term *psychotherapy* refers to the process that is used by mental health practitioners to help clients work through their problems. Often referred to as "talk therapy", there are many forms of psychotherapy and these will be addressed in chapter four. Psychotherapists are those professionals who assist people in dealing with their mental health issues—there are many different types of professionals in this area, such as psychiatrists, psychologists, social workers, marriage and family therapists, professional counselors, and psychiatric social workers, and others; these will be reviewed in chapter three.

Psychopharmacology

Psychopharmacology refers to the use of prescription medications to treat mental health disorders and conditions. The term psychotropic is often used to describe a large category of drugs for treating mental health conditions. These drugs include antidepressants, narcotics, stimulants, tranquilizers, and others. Although psychotropic drugs are sometimes prescribed by medical doctors to treat disorders without the use of psychotherapy, the use of these drugs in conjunction with psychotherapy has been found to be more effective than just the drug treatment alone. Of course, medications carry the risk of side effects which can sometimes complicate psychological disorders. Further elaborations on psychopharmacology will be examined in our discussion on psychotherapeutic treatment methods in chapter four.

Mental Health System

The *mental health system* as defined by the World Health Organization (WHO), "comprises all organizations, institutions, and resources whose primary purpose is to produce actions whose primary purpose is to improve mental health" (WHO, 2016, p.105). It is a subsystem of the general health care system and includes the institutions, policies, financing operations, treatments, and structures, that supports the provision of mental health services. It often refers to government (primarily state) operated facilities and programs, but we will use the "system" approach to include all providers and programs, including those that are privately administered. Mental health services include hospitalization, in-patient services, out-patient services, intensive out-patient treatment, day treatment programs, specialized community treatment, psychoeducation, and crisis intervention. Mental health case management refers to the provision of services in the mental health system through the referral to the appropriate organizations and programs within the system. Due to the emphasis of this book on the entire mental health system as well as its component parts, more information will be provided in chapter six.

Mental Health Advocacy

Advocacy refers to the representation of the needs and concerns of people or groups who lack a voice in achieving their rights. It involves the use of persuasion in that people, primarily policy holders, must be convinced of the legitimacy of their cause. It also involves emotional and psychological factors as these topics tend to stir deeply rooted feelings (Wilks, 2012). Often advocacy involves political elements as attention to the concerns of the advocacy "partners" have policy implications. Advocating for the mentally ill is a necessary and just cause, as will be discussed in chapter seven.

Therapeutic Substructure

Another term—*therapeutic substructure*—will be introduced in this work to examine the complex of cultural attitudes, beliefs, and historical background that supports ideas about the therapeutic alliance between therapist and client and the institutions upon which that alliance is built. It is the foundation that supports the buildings, diagnostic classification and procedures, treatment modalities, psychotherapy professions, funding sources, psychopharmacology, related systems, programs and resources for advocacy, and all other parts of the mental health apparatus that has been created by humans to address mental illness. It undergirds the hospitals, clinics, diagnostic manual, practice degrees and licensure (the "instrumental", or task-oriented part of the system) and consists of the nurturing, healing components of humanity (the "expressive" component).

The therapeutic substructure consists of the basic human need to assist those who are in pain, including the pain that comes from the stigma of being different. It is comprised of the emotional foundations that drive the system of mental health. It is the non-material culture of values and beliefs that serves as the foundation that supports the tangible material culture of the mental health enterprise.

This substructure contains the cultural understandings and responses to mental illness, such as etiology (what causes it), diagnosis (how we classify it), and practice (what we do to alleviate it), as well as policy (how we plan to institutionalize it). The substructure is dependent upon the history of mental health as a guide for the future. We make changes by reimaging and reimagine by looking closely beneath the surface. This concept will be used throughout the work to explain the cultural underpinnings of the other parts of the mental health system covered in the book.

CONCLUSION

The purpose of their book to explore the issue of mental illness and the mental health system that has been developed to deal with it. It provides information on this system in the hope that we reimagine the system that exists to help people working in therapeutic alliance with the mentally ill.

This text takes a sociological view of the mental health system by stepping back from the more technical aspects of mental illness and viewing the system. The term madness is used to provide context to the periods it was used and to show the changes in the treatment of the mentally ill. While changes in this treatment have taken place through the use of imagination, readers are asked to reimagine the mental health system through new dialogues and conversations that create this reimagining.

Any good analysis provides definitions for its key terms. Definitions for mental, health, mental illness, psychopathology, addictive disorder, mental health institutions, mental health diagnosis, psychotherapy, psychopharmacology, mental health system, and mental health advocacy were addressed, as well as another concept—the therapeutic substructure. These will be key concerns throughout the text which are necessary in understanding mental health as an active system with many working parts.

Chapter 2

A SHORT HISTORY OF MENTAL ILLNESS AND ITS TREATMENT

"by misunderstanding the past, we also misunderstand the present."
(Torrey & Miller, 2001, p. 3)

THE EARLIEST UNDERSTANDINGS OF "MADNESS"

Societies throughout history have attempted to understand the reasons people suffer from mental illness. They have also varied in their responses to the behaviors that resulted from these illnesses, actions that constituted violations of those societies' norms. The earliest known attributions to what we now consider mental illness involved the perceived existence of supernatural forces, in other words, demonic entities. Spiritual assumptions were used to explain bizarre and unexplainable behaviors in many ancient societies, including Egyptian, Greek and Roman, Asian, and early Christian societies. Though all believed in spiritual intervention by demons into the lives of the citizens, the causes were different in some respects, as well as the treatments.

The wrath of Yahweh upon the bad behavior of Egyptians is well documented in the Hebrew Bible as was manifest in plagues of different types, physical maladies, and death. Also documented was the occasional turning of prophets into madmen, devoid of their previous rationality (Scull, 2015). In antiquity the idea of healing resulted from a belief in magic. Amulets were thought to provide a powerful force in deterring evil spirits in early Egypt and these charms usually possessed the image of celestial bodies or sacred animals (Bromberg, 1959). Writings from ancient Egypt suggest that the treatment of people with mental illness consisted more of the "driving out" or "destroying" the disease rather than any attempts we would recognize today to treat or alleviate the symptoms of mental illness. While the Egypt of this period, sometimes called "the golden age", was touted for its high degree of civilization, its treatment of the mentally ill and idealized by some (such as 19th century French mental health reformer Phillipe Pinel), it was less than ideal in its treatment of those thought to be possessed by the plague of mental illness (Deutsch, 1949).

The deities in the mythology of ancient Greece who normally mingled with humans, occasionally caused them to be driven mad by the possession by demons; this theme was a major part of Greek writings, thus a salient part of Greek culture (Scull, 2015). This was not the only explanation in early Greece, however. Herodotus, a historian, posited two possible reasons for people acting erratically—an intervention by the gods or the existence of some internally produced disease, a dual-purpose explanation that came to be the common understanding of mental illness in the early Greek and Roman world. Many are familiar with the humoral theory proposed by early Greek physician Hippocrates (who disputed the spiritual causes of disease and for whom the Hippocratic Oath is named); according to the humoral theory all health conditions are created by the effects on the "four humors" of the body—blood, phlegm, yellow bile, and black bile (Rosen, 1968; Scull, 2015). Mental disease was especially correlated to black bile which, in large amounts would contribute to melancholia (today referred to as depression) (Rosen, 1968).

In early Christianity, some forms of what would today be considered mental illness were attributed to a "good madness", which happened when God intervened into the lives of prophets, religious visionaries, and holy innocents to carry out a divine directive. However, many people whose behavior or thoughts appeared erratic were believed to be possessed by the devil—a good example is the treatment of people whose actions made them suspect of being witches (Porter, 2002). It should be noted that while some of the people accused of witchcraft in Europe, and later the United States were mentally ill, the clear majority were not and were simply caught up in the new governmental and religious apparatus that was set up to induce conformity in a time that was filled with fear and uncertainty (Rosen, 1968). The witch craze in England eventually subsided around 1650 (Porter, 2002) but would also erupt in America in the same century with the executions of people suspected of demonic possession. The fear of witches, which also occurred in the American colonies, shines light on how behavior deemed bizarre can ignite fears that can have momentous consequences.

There are some similarities in how mental illness and illness generally were viewed in the East. Our knowledge of the ancient Chinese responses is somewhat sketchy, but we can determine the Eastern societies made less of a distinction between physical and mental disorders than their Western counterparts. While they also believed in spiritual explanations for illness to some extent—particularly in the form of the improper actions of past lives, demons and ghosts, fate, and cosmic irregularity—they also considered problems associated with exposure to the elements and imbalances that occurred within the body (the yin and yang of Taoist thought). In South Asia, Ayurvedic medical thought held that illness occurred with an imbalance of body fluids (like the Hippocratic humors) and that a realignment was needed to heal the body (Scull, 2015).

The global historical context of the treatment of mentally ill people is extremely complex, much more than the digest provided above. The reader, if interested in this field, is advised to consult the many books and articles that exist on this subject. They provide some insight into the current treatment of the mentally ill. As an old saying goes, "you don't know where you are going until you know where you've been". It behooves people interested in the advocacy of the mentally ill to learn more of this history. America's treatment of the mentally ill is equally interesting and equally illustrative of phases, and we will review it now.

THE EVOLUTION OF THE MENTAL HEALTH SYSTEM IN AMERICA

Kurtz (1987) has posited six different phases or movements that have occurred in the mental health field in the United States. These stages acknowledge some degree of success in the progression of mental health treatment but note the system continually was met with setbacks—hospital overcrowding, economizing, a scarcity of resources, and later neglect—at each phase. The cycle, however, can be broken and greater success can be achieved if policy makers today can closely analyze the mistakes that were made in these movements of the past and be willing to act to correct present and future policy approaches regarding the treatment of mental illness. We will now view these stages.

Colonial Period

The first of these stages begins in colonial America, where people who exhibited signs of mental illness were, as in many other parts of the world and mentioned previously, assumed to be possessed by demons. Many of them were subjected to common forms of punishment, torture, and death (such as the rack, the stake, or the gallows), incarcerated in dungeons, or, if dangerousness was not determined, they were allowed the wander the streets with no assistance (people in this category were often called Toms o' Bedlam). Although some attempts were made to eradicate religious explanations of mental illness in the 17th century, the fear of witchcraft was universal in the colonies, as it had been earlier in Europe. In some cases, they were taken to the Church, so the clergy could attempt to exorcise the demons. The witchcraft scare in Salem, Massachusetts from 1691 to 1692 reflected this perspective and resulted in the deaths of 20 people and the torture of 200 others. The next year the governor of the Massachusetts Colony released all people incarcerated for suspicion of witchcraft (Deutsch, 1949).

Moral Treatment Movement

The second phase, commonly referred to as the moral treatment movement of the late eighteenth and early nineteenth centuries, occurred when reformers such as France's Phillippe Pinel, a physician, symbolically ordered the chains removed from hospitalized mental patients, and institutionalized humane reforms for the mentally ill. In England, William Tuke instituted Quaker ideals and advocated for reforms for the cruel treatment received by patients in British asylums. And in America, the physician Benjamin Rush created the country's first hospital designed under the auspices of the moral treatment movement for the mentally ill patients housed there. Hospitals specifically designed for the mentally ill began in America in 1773 in Williamsburg, Virginia and followed slowly in the 1800s by institutions in Kentucky, Massachusetts, New York, and other states. Another major reformer of this movement was Dorothea Dix whose advocacy for the mentally ill resulted in the founding of 32 public mental hospitals that offered moral treatment for those hospitalized there.

Although the plans for these institutions in this second stage was to remain small, an increase in an immigrant population, rapid changes wrought by urbanization, and a growing number of disabled elderly patients resulted in the erection of state hospitals that were much larger than planned; these behemoth institutions became overcrowded and care for the mentally ill regressed (Kurtz, 1987). The result of mass institutionalization in these asylums was not only overcrowding but also patient neglect, malnourishment, and barbaric "treatments" such as lobotomies, and various shock treatments. Managing this massive system with little financial support was impossible and the mental health system was forced to change (Joffe, 2016).

Mental Hygiene Movement

The third stage, the mental hygiene movement of the early 1900s, sought to improve the conditions that had degenerated in the moral treatment phase. Reformer and former mental patient Clifford Beers, who had experienced firsthand the problems of the institutions, published a classic book *A Mind that Found Itself* in 1908, a work that advocated reorganization of the hospitals and the creation of state mental health associations

(Kurtz, 1987; Fancher, 1995). Rather than focus on mental illness prevention, Beers was convinced by the nation's foremost psychiatrist Adolph Meyer to instead concentrate on advocating "mental hygiene" (Fancher, 1995). It was during this stage that child guidance clinics were formed, utilizing the skills of social workers in their expertise of children and families. These child guidance clinics had grown in number to over 600 by the late 1950s and would provide the framework for what would become community mental health programs (Kurtz, 1987).

Community Mental Health Movement

The fourth of these phases occurred shortly after World War II and ushered in a new era in mental health policies and initiatives. The National Institute of Mental Health (NIMH) was authorized in 1946 through the National Mental Health Act, the first important federal mental health legislation. Emphasized during this period from a treatment perspective were:

- brief interventions
- crisis strategies
- diagnosis
- prevention
- the training of mental health personnel (Kurtz, 1987).

President John F. Kennedy addressed mental health in his "bold new approach" that sought to fund a national program of community mental health care; in this effort over 760 community centers were created over the next two decades. Provided in this directive were several types of services:

- inpatient
- outpatient
- crisis
- partial hospitalization
- consultation/education

These became overtaxed as the period of institutionalization progressed and the influx of severely mentally ill patients, who were originally housed in institutions, entered the system (Kurtz, 1987).

Deinstitutionalization

Deinstitutionalization, the fifth movement, is well known in the history of American mental health policy and has been described by one scholar as one of the nation's largest experiments (Torrey, 1997). The activism that characterized American society in the late 1960s and early 1970s eventually found its way to the treatment of the hospitalized mentally ill in America. Legal decisions promoting the least restrictive treatment environments for mental health patients resulted in the discharge of many chronically ill patients into the communities, who were unable to support them. The optimism of the prior period was dampened with this overwhelming dictate and mental health programs tried in vain to accommodate it (Kurtz, 1987). This period has been referred to by one scholar as "decarceration"—when people who were housed in mental hospitals and juvenile reformatories were released into communities who were then charged with the responsibility of providing community-based services (Scull, 1977).

Deinstitutionalization was brought about by six other factors (Joffe, 2016):

1. The media exposure of the deteriorating hospital conditions and treatment of patients
2. New medications that were able to provide some degree of symptom relief and behavioral maintenance
3. Financing for community-based centers
4. Insurance availability for inpatient mental health coverage in general hospitals
5. Federal legislation that prompted stricter involuntary commitment laws

The new deinstitutionalization measures failed for the same reason mass institutionalization failed—lack of financial planning for these dramatic changes (Joffe, 2016).

Decade of Scarcity

The decade of scarcity, the sixth phase identified, was characterized by the fiscal cutbacks of Ronald Reagan's administration in the 1980s. Governmental regulations were removed from many mental health programs and states were forced to fend for themselves. Since the chronically mentally ill are often unable to pay for billable services; this created major changes in the system (Kurtz, 1987). The focus on fiscal responsibility and a desire to shift the authority to the states occurred in tandem with a more punitive approach to crime and a willingness to support limited mental health programming. The easing of standards not only in mental health, but also crime and homelessness was the national zeitgeist. The stakeholders in this movement consisted of an unusual mix of fiscal conservatives, law and order Republicans, and liberal activists (Thomas, 1998).

Criminalization of the Mentally Ill

If we were to bring the current mental health situation into a more contemporary analysis that updates the stage model listed above, we should mention the phenomena of the criminalization of the mentally ill—this reflects the fact that the mentally ill often commit nuisance crimes such as disorderly conduct or ordinance violations, with no intent to indulge in major criminal behavior. In addition, "mercy bookings" occur in which the police charge the mentally ill for petty offenses, so they can receive food, lodging, and some degree of care—well-meaning officers then contribute to the problem as jails are normally not equipped to handle the mental health needs of inmates (Joffe, 2016). Adopting a social constructionist approach, criminalization of the mentally ill suggests the framing of mental illness changed from the care of the sick to the punishment of deviants (see Erikson and Erikson 2008).

While the idea of mentally ill persons being directed into the jail and prison system is certainly not new, the mentally ill currently are highly overrepresented in the prison population. What is known as the "hydraulic hypothesis" is the idea that there will always be a portion of the mentally ill that will be housed in some institutional setting. The release of patients from mental institutions during the deinstitutionalization phase resulted in an influx of the mentally ill into correctional facilities, creating a situation that needed remedy. A strategy was developed to attend to the problem in the form of mental health courts and the first of these appeared in Florida in 1997. These courts have personnel that are specifically trained to work with mentally ill offenders and to divert them from correctional settings to therapeutic ones, easing the burden on both the criminal justice and mental health systems. While there were only four of these courts in 1997, there are over 300 today, existing in most almost of the states (Joffe, 2016).

It is perhaps beneficial to engage in a more detailed examination of the major historical events that represent the treatment of the mentally ill. While a stage model as the one presented above is helpful, there is no sharp delineation between the periods and there exists some overlap. We will now view one of the most noteworthy aspects of the history of the mental health system in the United States—the evolution of the mental hospital.

FROM LUNATIC ASYLUM TO THE MODERN MENTAL HOSPITAL

Many people are familiar with the term Bedlam, which normally denotes chaos and disorder. The term is a reference to a London asylum dating back to the 13th century called Bethlam Royal Hospital, which picked up the moniker Bedlam, which is now synonymous with extreme confusion and insanity. The idea of institutions of the insane has become the source of much lore and has created visions of laughing or screaming patients locked together in inhumane conditions and is often depicted in art, movies, and television shows as an example of what can happen when a society collapses upon itself. Mental hospitals in America also have an interesting history from the first one established in the 18th century to the present.

In colonial America prior to the founding of the health hospitals, the mentally ill were housed in many different settings including the homes of family members or themselves, the homes of local doctors, incarceration facilities (called gaols), workhouses, poorhouses, or living on the streets or in the countryside (Talbott, 1978) with other dependent "outcasts"—the homeless, beggars, the disabled, and the elderly (Zwelling, 1985). In 1752, the first mental ward of a general hospital was opened at the Pennsylvania Hospital (Talbott, 1978) and in 1833, the first state asylum was founded in Worchester, Massachusetts. As noted earlier, the first public hospital in the United States reserved for the mentally ill was founded in Williamsburg, Virginia in 1773 (Talbott, 1978; Zwelling, 1985)—reflecting the sign of the times, this hospital was named the Public Hospital for Persons of Insane and Disordered Minds.

With the advent of asylums in the United States, many American physicians were employed in the running of these institutions. Prior to the late 1800s, doctors in America were not well educated, well trained, well respected, or even well paid—normally making only general laborer's wages. The mental hospitals provided much better pay and more prestige, less than their European counterparts but much more than they had previously known. These "doctors for the insane" (Fancher, 1995) created the nation's first medical specialty—insanity. Another term for these early psychiatrists was "mad doctor" or "alienist", which was not necessarily used in a derogatory manner at the time.

Mental hospitals continued to appear in the 19th century, many of them going by the name asylum or lunatic hospital. The more commonly used term asylum is derived from Latin and means "no right of seizure", referring to the fact that these were places where people who acted in a fashion evidencing mental illness were protected (that is, given "asylum") from criminal prosecution (Calloway, 2007). The first such hospital to accept indigent patients was the Eastern Kentucky Lunatic Asylum, which was established in 1822. During this century, the states continued to provide different types of charitable services—in the form of poorhouses, orphanages, general hospitals, and mental hospitals, until the state governments began assuming more responsibility in this area. Later, the counties would adopt some of these social welfare functions, but the states were still prominent in the administration of the mental hospitals (Deutsch, 1949). Conditions of the late 19th century hospitals continued to deteriorate, and the abuses were well known, and in some cases exaggerated. Overcrowding in the state institutions continued until around 1955 when the entrance of new psychotropic drugs, policy decisions concerning outpatient treatment (community mental health), and funding initiates for the mentally ill treatment in for the elderly in nursing homes, culminated in the deinstitutionalization movement (Talbott, 1978). Deinstitutionalization, as noted earlier, created the community mental health model that continues to dominate mental health care in America.

Curious about the unexplained increase of mental illness that occurred in the United States, Canada, England, and Ireland from the mid-eighteenth century to the mid-twentieth centuries, an increase that could only be described as an "invisible epidemic", Torrey and Miller (2001) cast doubt on the so-called "lumber room thesis" that posits the increase and later overcrowding of patients in asylums was due to the phenomenon of available spaces offering opportunities to fill them. The authors refuted the numerous explanations that have been posited to explain this increase—such as asylums being used as dumping groups for family members; that they were repositories for the odd, eccentric, and generally deviant; that the asylums were welcomed in the community by citizens willing to have their taxes increased, etc. and concluded that the problems might be related to changes in civilization, notably urbanization and individualization, that can create changes in mental functioning. We will soon observe how theorists such as Erich Fromm viewed society itself as becoming increasingly insane. Torrey and Miller (2001) explain how, in addition to the stress hypotheses that have been so commonly considered a corollary to mental illness, it is possible that changes in diet, alcohol availability, modern toxins, infectious agents, and access to medical care could be factors that have influenced the "epidemic" of mental illness since the nineteenth century.

As with the global history of mental illness, it is important to understand the national history as well, warts and all. As the movement model suggests, we must understand each of the stages we have experienced to ascertain a better course of action in the treatment of the mentally ill. There will always be social and political changes and realities that will redirect this course, but we will at least be prepared and know how to direct our advocacy. An understanding of even the darkest eras in our treatment of the mentally ill is important—even the phenomenon we refer to as eugenics.

THE DARK SHADOW OF EUGENICS

The dark period of American history at the turn of the 20th century known as the eugenics movement established the involuntary sterilization of certain groups. This movement was based on the premise that certain people—primarily criminal offenders, the impoverished, the mentally ill, and the developmentally disabled—would contribute to the ruin of society if allowed to reproduce (Rosen, 1968). This was a cause championed decades earlier by Britain's Francis Galton to rid his country of undesirables. Eugenics had at its core the philosophy of social Darwinism and reflected issues of race, ethnicity, class, nativity, and other characteristics that were of a concern in a rapidly changing society experiencing an influx of foreign immigrants.

By the 1920s, the practice of sterilizing the mentally ill was increasingly popular; this was a practice that continued until the 1960s, with the idea that "undesirables", including the mentally ill, should not reproduce as their progeny might also have the same afflictions and thus be a blight on society. Supreme Court Justice Oliver Wendell Holmes famously quoted "three generations of imbeciles are enough", in his argument in 1927's case Buck v. Bell reflecting this idea (Joffe, 2016). Ostensibly, eugenics was carried out to create a better society, and one could realize that proponents seemed to be promoting an attempt to interject scientific reasoning—at least based on scientific understandings of their time—rather than basing the behavior of these groups on individual moral failings. However, the extreme cruelty exhibited to what we would now consider "the other" is truly amazing and the undercurrents of bigotry are obvious. We would be well-served to look beyond our own prejudices and realize the way to help others is to not judge and certainly not to take actions that would harm them.

THE POST-WORLD WAR II ERA

As noted earlier, after the Second World War, it became clear the old state hospitals were becoming too old and costly to maintain (Johnson, 1990). In the 1950s, a joint commission of the American Medical Association and the American Psychiatric Association investigated the mental health system and recommended, among other things, a refurbishing of the state hospital system, however, they wanted the institutions to be smaller. At a secondary level, there was a call to establish prevention services and to create an outpatient system of mental health care. President Kennedy took office in 1961, and soon thereafter he created the Community Mental Health Centers Act with the intention that the Federal government would provide funding for the startup of what would soon be called community mental health or community psychology programs. Federal funding for the initiative decreased significantly in the 1970s. The program was initially based on the ideas of psychiatrists, psychologists, and sociologists; however, it would become more controlled by the medical field, legislative agendas, and the complex interrelationships between the Federal government and the many local governments that directly administered community mental health; this system became complex and convoluted (Levine, 1981). The model is still in use and provides many outpatient mental health services.

In the early years of the twentieth century, prior to the community mental health system, not all people who were experiencing emotional problems were receiving treatment in hospitals—some were being seen by private therapists, primarily psychiatrists who were M.D.'s with additional training in mental illness. Talk therapy was available to some people, those whose mental health problems were not severe enough to require hospitalization, and who were able to afford it. As in Europe, many psychiatrists in America were using Sigmund Freud's psychoanalysis in their work with patients. Psychoanalysis is both a theory and a treatment method that believes that the source of mental illness lies in the anxiety existing deep in the recesses of the mind. In the treatment program, counseling is needed to bring these thoughts to consciousness through such strategies as free association and dream analysis. Psychoanalytic outpatient therapy was lengthy and expensive, thus only the well-to-do could afford it, others had to deal with their problems on their own, or enter the hospital (Engel, 2008). So, in the early decades of the twentieth century, some patients were hospitalized and others who were able to afford it, received outpatient therapy, of which the growing methodology called psychoanalysis was often a part. Psychoanalysis continued to be a major force after the early post-war period, but its preeminence would wane in coming decades.

After World War II, major changes took place in psychotherapy. The numerous military inductees that were brought into testing centers exhibited a host of mental problems that greatly concerned the federal government. In addition, the effects of the war on the soldiers' emotional health were considerable. Therefore, psychiatrists were enlisted to assist in dealing with these issues, however, there were not enough of these specialists to meet the need. The services of psychiatric social workers began to be enlisted as well. Social workers, who were primarily women, were trained in dealing with clients lives in their social context, and their interpersonal skills were beneficial in dealing with this often-traumatized population. Social workers were also trained in psychoanalysis during this period (which shows the primacy of this therapy in the nascent field of social work), but the actual treatment was (or at least was supposed to be) performed by the doctors. As the war progressed, additional assistance was needed, therefore, psychologists were also recruited to assist in delivering mental health services to military personnel. Prior to this time psychologists were primarily tasked with providing psychological assessments for the military, schools, and corporations as clinical psychology was still embryonic; these scientists had to adjust to counseling duties instead of their more quantitative pursuits. Psychoanalysis, so important to the psychiatrists and social workers, was not eschewed by the more scientifically oriented psychologists at mid-century. Conflict occasionally existed between these groups (as it still does), but these three types of mental health practitioners—psychiatrists, psychologists, and social workers—became the outpatient mental health treatment providers at mid-twentieth century (Engel, 2008). The psychiatrists continued to maintain the reins over the team, however.

New drugs began appearing on the scene to help alleviate the symptoms of various emotional issues and many psychiatrists returned to medicine, cutting some of their ties to psychoanalysis as the century progressed. The role of psychiatrists as the primary practitioners in mental health treatment continued to decline after 1970 as the role of social workers and clinical psychologists continued to increase. The latter two groups continued to develop their fields as the effects of deinstitutionalization changed the landscape of mental health in America (Engel, 2008). Marriage and family therapists also appeared on the scene after World War II and emphasized the interactions between people in the family and explored how past family influences affect thoughts and behavior and contribute to some of the emotional problems people face. As many psychiatrists had desired to remove patients from families they considered dysfunctional, family therapists believed positive change could better be achieved by working with the family as a unit—ironically, many of these early family therapists were trained in psychoanalytic psychiatry. Starting in the 1950s and 1960s, researchers began to investigate families in treatment and the field continued to grow (Barker, 1986).

The 1970s was considered by one theorist of culture (Lasch, 1979) as representing a "culture of narcissism" in which perhaps society itself suffered from insanity. Therefore, while the focus of therapeutic treatment in the 1960s was on the saving of society itself, the next decade focused on people trying to save their individual psyches. Humanistic models such as person-centered therapy and gestalt theory, which provided an intense focus on individual growth and happiness, became attractive forms of therapy because of this focus on the self. Some "unique" therapeutic techniques that became popular in this period were "primal" models that directed patients to deprive themselves of normal human indulgences, "rebirthing" techniques that involve imagining oneself going through the traumatic process of birth, and dance movement strategies that induce thoughts and feelings through dance; today these are often lumped together under the name body psychotherapy (Totten, 2003).

Drug therapies continued into the 1980s and the antidepressant Prozac became the magic pill of the era, not only prescribed by psychiatrists but also general physicians and internists. Psychotherapies became more eclectic and much shorter in duration, driven in part by drug therapy and in part by the managed care system which sought to provide the cheapest and shortest treatment to control health care costs (Engel, 2008). Newer psychotherapies continued to appear prior the end of the 20th century such as emotion-centered theory, mindfulness models, solution-focused treatment, narrative therapy, and integrated models. Specialty areas such as trauma therapy, online therapy, and eye movement desensitization and reprocessing (EMDR) therapy also appeared. These therapies will be discussed in more length in the following chapter.

A particularly controversial treatment of this type involved the use of recovered memory techniques that sought to bring out of consciousness patient's recollections of child abuse (often sexual abuse) that were blocked; the problem of the fallibility of memory brought about lawsuits and restrictions on professional practice in the 1990s.

Under the administration of George W. Bush, the New Freedom Commission on Mental Health was created. This program produced an unfavorable analysis of the mental health system in place at that time as it related to how jails and prisons were housing large numbers of mentally ill inmates. Federal funding supported mental health courts and diversionary programs for the mentally ill in attempts to provide psychiatric services rather than incarceration (Erickson & Erickson, 2008).

A major issue in the mental health care field in the early part of the 21th century involves the funding of mental health care (and health care generally). A centerpiece of President Barack Obama's administration was the Patient Protection and American Healthcare Act (called the ACA or the more popular moniker "Obamacare"), which provided employee mandates and penalties for healthcare coverage and mental health coverage (Cutler, Sills, Svendsen, & Yeager, 2013). Donald Trump was elected President in 2016 and vowed to repeal and replace the ACA but did not get full support from Congress for the repeal. Currently, attempts for creating a new health care system is still being fought in Congress and could determine the fate of many in the mental health care system.

THE UNIQUE HISTORY OF THE TREATMENT OF ADDICTION

Substance abuse treatment is considered in this book on mental illness because in many ways the two disorders converge, as noted in the introductory chapter. Substance abuse is considered a mental disorder in the Diagnostic Manual of Mental Disorders (DSM)), many of the treatment methods are the same, and addiction often is a co-occurring condition with other mental health conditions. In addition, the idea that addiction is a disease is often considered in the same manner as biologically-supported mental illnesses. The history of the treatment of substance addictions in America is very rich and distinct among nations.

While alcohol had been a major part of American social life since colonial life, concerns later developed over the use of stronger spirits and excessive use, which was thought to be directly connected to a variety of social ills. Physician Benjamin Rush, who was also called the "father of psychiatry", mounted a campaign in the late eighteen-century to combat alcoholism and to promote abstinence from drinking. The coming years would see conflicts between those who supported temperance and those who wanted to drink. The "noble experiment" of prohibition in 1920 and its repeal in 1933 continued to shine a spotlight on alcohol and its consequences. The novel approach of self-help known as Alcoholics Anonymous (informally known as AA) began in 1935 which involved:

- attendance at meetings that were directed by members rather than non-professional staff;
- individual sponsorship;
- and a rigid protocol ("the twelve steps"),

all of which were utilized to promote total abstinence from drinking. AA became a prominent national model that is still in use today and spurred other popular programs such as Narcotics Anonymous (NA), and Cocaine Anonymous (CA). People addicted to alcohol and other drugs became seen as people whose behavior was beyond their control, which is quite a change from earlier considerations.

The idea for hospitals specifically created for alcohol addiction goes back at least to the early 19th century when Benjamin Rush proposed a "sober house". At mid-century, the plans were laid to create such hospitals, based on the mental asylum model but located in rural areas and focusing on what we now call recovery (Baumohl, 1990). The plan came to fruition in 1864 when the first such hospital, the New York Inebriate Asylum, was founded at a time when ideas about addiction had evolved from substance abuse as a personal failing to the concept of addiction as a disease. When key players sought to professionalize the field, they found some unlikely common ground with the temperance movement. These key figures opened several other hospitals, some of which offered treatment programs for other drugs of abuse such as the Walnut Lodge Hospital in Connecticut offering services for "alcohol and opium inebriates"; while some were specific to women (Lender & Martin, 1987). The inebriate asylums would end in the 1920s during the prohibition era and private hospitals were made available for the more affluent, causing addicts to return to the streets.

In 1960, E.M. Jellinek published *The Disease Concept of Alcoholism*, one of the most quoted but least read books in the field (White, 2014) which promoted the disease concept in a manner that was accepted by many lay people and professionals. This concept aligned well with the positions espoused in AA, therefore it became very popular; however, it was not without its detractors. The disease concept dates to at least the eighteenth century when Benjamin Rush posited the concept along with strategies to cure this disease. If substance abuse is indeed a disease, it is presumed that the cure should be sought in abstinence from the substance in conjunction with strong social supports to maintain sobriety.

Organizations called therapeutic communities were derived from a substance abuse program called Synanon, a support community for addicted people begun in 1958. These programs worked to return substance abusers to functional roles, accepted public funds, adhered to governmental guidelines, and staffed their programs with graduates of therapeutic communities. The programs, which resembled halfway houses (programs that housed people who were between incarceration and community) became popular in the 1960s and 1970s (White, 2014).

Substance abuse treatment (for all types of chemical substances, and later with behavioral disorders such as gambling) became very professionalized as new and emerging treatment types such as the famous "Minnesota model" appeared on the scene and grew in popularity. This program had its roots in the programs in the late 1940s and three of these are notable: an A-based short-term treatment facility called Pioneer House; a Minnesota farmhouse turned into an alcohol addiction retreat known as Hazelden that sought to correct a person's alcoholism before that person ended up losing everything; and a mental institution called Willmar Hospital that treated chronic alcoholics and worked from a new philosophy of addiction. The Hazelden facility branched out into other states and began publishing addictions-related pamphlets; it would eventually become the largest producer of self-help material in the world (White, 2014).

In the mid-1960s, a program called methadone maintenance began and sought to treat heroin addiction. Since there was no national drug treatment regime at the time, the field was open to new ideas, even controversial ones, and this program continues to exist today. What makes the program so controversial is that heroin users were given the drug methadone, which is also a highly addictive opioid. Methadone, however, doesn't create a "high" and enables users of other drugs to wean off their addiction and can assist with chronic pain. The drug's properties, which include tolerance and dependence, have been obviously met with negative reactions by some anti-drug advocates and those who believe in total abstinence from drugs (Kuhn, Swartzenwelder, & Wilson, 2008).

The 1980s saw a renewed focus on education-based substance abuse prevention programs such as first lady Nancy Reagan's "Just Say No program" in 1982 which consisted of a series of public services announcements; while well intended, it was not as effective as hoped. The Drug Abuse Resistance Education (known better as D.A.R.E.), began in 1983 as a coordinated effort between a police department and school district in Los Angeles that sought to provide life skills, resistance training, and self-esteem building to better refrain from drugs and violence; it later became a national model. While the original version of D.A.R.E. was found to be ineffective, it is hoped that newer models will provide better outcome data (Singh et al., 2011). Other schemes to keep young people away from drug abuse and other delinquencies such as "scared straight" programs that place the youngsters around hardened prison inmates, have produced mostly unsatisfactory results; popularized in a 1979 documentary (and decade later a TV series), the program was meant to scare young offenders straight to a prosocial lifestyle, but studies have shown that the program, along with its spin-offs, have been primarily found to be ineffective or even detrimental to encouraging a drug and crime free lifestyle (Klenowski, Bell, & Dodson, 2010; Royster, 2012).

The Johnson intervention, often just called an intervention, is a "tough love" strategy in which family members or other people close to someone addicted to drugs directly confront the user and threaten a loss of support unless in-patient treatment is completed. This treatment model became known nationally with the popularity of a TV reality show which began in the first decade of the new millennium. Although the idea of this tough love strategy became fashionable, the withdrawal of a user's support group makes the approach difficult for some relatives to carry out.

A substance use treatment model called "harm reduction" (Tatarsky & Marlett, 2010) started in Europe in the 1970s and developed in the 1990s in America. This format promotes controlled use of substances and is controversial in that it runs counter to the traditional twelve step propositions that provide that users must be abstinent in their use of substances before treatment can be effective; however, it has provided another way of understanding both addiction and its treatment. The model assumes that substance abuse is a reality (and a harmful one at that) and it is preferable to place a treatment emphasis on minimizing the harms, such as overdoses, HIV transmission, car accidents, instead of enforcing a strict zero tolerance of use. Adherents claim these types of programs are more effective than abstinence-based schemes (MacMaster, 2004; Lushin & Anastas, 2011).

Drug courts began in Florida in 1989 due to the influx of cocaine, crack and PCP (Dembo & Pacheco, 1999) and have spread to many areas of the country. This program, which specifically targets drug offenses with its specific treatment focus, has shown some early signs of promise in the first two decades of the 21st century. It is expected that the use of these drug courts, much like their mental health counterparts, will continue to grow unless state drug policies require a different course.

America has experienced several different "waves" of addiction scares dating back to the Progressive Era's cocaine scare. After World War II, many people in the 1960s and 1970s were concerned about the increasing use of drugs by young people. There have been many times since then that these waves have caught the attention of a large part of American society such as the PCP "angel dust" scare of the late 1970s, the crack cocaine scare of the 1980s, and the methamphetamine concerns of the 1990s, resulting in what some consider "moral panics" (Acker, 2002), which are widespread, but often irrational, fears. Recently, a concern over prescription opioid abuse has been dominating the national news and is unlikely to be considered a moral panic as approximately 2 million Americans abused and were addicted to opioids (especially Methadone, Oxycodone, and Hydrocodone) in 2015. A major concern with opioid abuse is the high level of death by overdose—over 15,000 people died by overdose in 2015 (CDC, n.d.). Since these drugs are prescribed and used for pain management, the issue of abuse is certainly problematic. And the past abuse of prescribed opioids is the highest risk factor for addiction to heroin, which accounted for another 13,000 overdose deaths in 2015 (CDC, n.d.).

CONCLUSION

A sociohistorical approach reveals that religion and spirituality were key contributors to understandings of mental illness and mental disorders in many early societies though the specific assumptions and interventions varied. There have been stages in the evolution of the mental health system in America—the colonial period, moral treatment, mental hygiene movement, community health program, the action known as deinstitutionalization, the decade of scarcity, and the criminalization of the mentally ill. It is important to review and understand these stages as they provide the cultural understandings of the substructure that drive us to seek positive changes in the field of mental health. Without a reflection of our rich history and the therapeutic substructure that contributed to it, an understanding such as this cannot occur.

The sociohistorical approach also traces early methods of treating the mentally ill from their placement in what were termed lunatic asylums, which was a change from housing them in almshouses and jails. The eugenics movement of the twentieth century illustrated another attempt to control mental illness in America. After World War II, strategies were developed to create a better mental health system and paved the way for deinstitutionalization.

The war caused a new cadre of mental health workers to assist psychiatrists in some cases and to compete with them in others. Psychoanalysis, which had reigned as the supreme method of treatment began to falter at mid-twentieth century. Psychopharmacological treatments entered the scene and have continued to increase in importance. The recent introduction of mental health courts offers a potential counter to what has been termed the criminalization of mental illness.

Addiction and its treatment also has a long and interesting history with an assortment of responses to "waves" and "scares". Treatment programs for substance addiction have involved some questionable strategies, but many have remained. The disease model of addiction reflects an ideological position that has transformed our understandings of addiction, however, it has always been subject to challenge. Likewise, treatment approaches that stress abstinence has sustained critique, recently in the form of harm reduction approaches. Like mental health courts, drug courts have been instituted that seek to provide more effective services for addicted people involved in criminal activity.

Chapter 3

THE DSM, MENTAL HEALTH DISORDERS, AND THE PSY-PROFESSIONALS

> "I was told that the great specialist had admitted to friends of his that he had altered his treatment of neurasthenia since reading 'The Yellow Wallpaper'...It was not intended to drive people crazy, but to save people from being driven crazy, and it worked."
>
> (Charlotte Perkins Gilman, 1913)

THE DIAGNOSTIC AND STATISTICAL MANUAL OF MENTAL DISORDERS (DSM)

Since most mental illnesses are considered conditions that can be treated, or at least have symptoms ameliorated, there has been a need to find a way to diagnose the problems. The DSM (Diagnostic and Statistical Manual of Mental Disorders) is the official guide for mental health diagnosis and its impression upon the mental health field has been immense, especially regarding the conditions that are considered mental disorders and the people whose job it is to treat them. The DSM was not the first document to attempt to categorize mental disorders, however, as we shall see. Diagnosis refers to the identification of diseases or disorders (in this case mental disorders) by careful observation of the disorders' characteristics. A successful diagnosis provides a basis for prognosis and is assumed to be the beginning of the process of treatment. Diagnosis relies upon a classification scheme—an arrangement of several characteristics into a cluster which creates a distinct type of disorder. The related term nosology refers to this type of classification system.

Mental health diagnosis, as with other types, requires an assessment which involves intense questioning and recording of the person's situation based on presenting symptomology, impairment of functioning, and duration of the problem. It also requires judgement on the part of the diagnostician to decide the appropriate classification of the disorder (Mirowsky & Ross, 1989).

The diagnosis process is completed using these four steps:

1. Assessing symptoms, impairment, and duration of the condition
2. "Splitting" the amounts of symptomology in two categories—those that met diagnostic criteria and those that do not
3. "Totting up" those met/unmet criteria that merge together symptoms, impairment, and duration
4. Ruling out other potential categories (Miroswsky & Ross, 1989).

Diagnosis is an important part of the overall system of mental health service provision with a fascinating history of evolving nosologies. We will now look at a brief history of events leading up to the DSM, including its predecessors.

A SHORT HISTORY OF MENTAL HEALTH DIAGNOSIS

Before the DSM

Attempts to adequately diagnose "madness" have a long history. In the 19th century, observations of various constitutional (or bodily) features produced some interesting strategies for diagnosis; possibly the best known of these is phrenology, the study of the bumps on the head. This diagnostic "procedure" rested on the understanding that the brain contains parts that provide different cognitive functions. By feeling the skull, one could ascertain if someone had an excess or a dearth of a certain characteristic, by the existence of an extruding or depressed bump. While the feeling of head bumps became very popular in the early 1800s as sort of a parlor game, its use as a mental assessment had died out by mid-century. The fact that phrenology attracted celebrated writers of the time, including Mark Twain, who apparently had conflicting feelings about the practice (Gribben, 1972), attests to its popularity. Other constitutional assessments sought to find a link between mental functioning and the body. Though now regarded as pseudo-science, these attempts were worthwhile in that they brought us closer to an understanding of mental illness and its classification.

Classification of items does not represent a static image of reality, but rather a representation that is based on human experiences and observations which are relevant to historical time and place, as well as other social and political factors; in other words, mental health diagnoses are not as firm and fixed as we often think. At mid-nineteenth century, psychiatrists had little use for nosologies of mental illness, at least as they relate to clinical practice, as they doubted their practical utility. They did, however, understand how the collection of statistical information could provide basic principles of mental illness that affect patient recovery, assist in advocacy of issues, and add support for legitimizing the profession. Statistics require classification activity to make sense of the data and put it to practical use. An early nineteenth century class scheme involved only two categories—idiocy/imbecility (we would consider neurodevelopmental disorders today) and mania/dementia (neurocognitive conditions) (Grob, 1991). A series of events would promote the evolution of mental health diagnosis.

The nineteenth century saw further attempts at a mental health classification system and came up with a few categories of mental illness, however, these categories were meant to be used for demographic rather than nosological reasons. Knowing that they lacked any scientific evidence of the etiology, or cause of mental disorders, they were reticent to produce a true classification system for clinical purposes. There were many social variables such as a specific client's relationship concerns, educational attainment, environmental issues, and occupational problems in the field of psychiatry that made such a classification system difficult (Grob, 1991).

Interestingly, the United States census is linked to the development of a mental illness classification as it provided demographic information which was collected in part to ascertain the effects of immigration in a rapidly changing country in the 19th century. During the moral treatment period, the 1840 census had a classification system based on mental health and had the categories of sane and idocity/insanity (psychosis). The 1880 census had seven categories:

1. Dementia
2. Dipsomania (alcohol addiction)
3. Mania
4. Melancholia (depression)
5. Monomania (comparable to today's obsessive-compulsive disorder)
6. Paresis (bodily weakness due to nerve damage) (LaBruzza, 1997).

Fears of the effects of native-born Americans mixing with immigrants considered racially and ethnically inferior produced a major concern for many in the majority and would eventually lead to marital restrictions, segregation of the mentally ill, and eugenics activity (Grob, 1991).

As the century waned, there was a renewed interest in mental illness nosology. Emil Kraepelin, a German psychiatrist, undertook a massive data gathering effort from mental health patients at his clinic, in search of common symptomology from which to create a classification system (Grob, 1991). Kraepelin is often given credit for producing, albeit in elementary form, the first effort to diagnose mental conditions in 1883 when he published a small textbook which became known as the *Short Textbook of Psychiatry*, which would develop in eight revisions, being published until 1927. The *Textbook* was not intended to be a comprehensive classification of mental disorders as we know today but it did identify two distinct forms of mental illness—manic depression insanity, today known as bipolar disorder, and dementia praecox, currently named schizophrenia (Malik & Beutler, 2002).

In 1918, the National Center for Mental Hygiene developed the lengthy titled *Statistical Manual for the Use of Institutions for the Insane* as the first standardized classified guide, which went through ten revised editions until the 1940s (Grob, 1991; Clegg, 2012). In 1920, based on the *Statistical Manual*, the U.S. Census began reporting the number of people in mental institutions. The new nosology was not accepted by everyone, however; one of the biggest opponents was esteemed American psychiatrist Adolf Meyer, who rejected the Kraepelin-influenced system, encouraging his medical students to follow suit (Grob, 1991). The *Statistical Manual* focused on biological causes and features of mental illness, which was the standard perspective until World War II. Many psychiatrists during the war rejected the biological orientation of the previous decades and accepted the increasingly influential psychoanalytic approach, heralded by Sigmund Freud (this treatment theory and method will be mentioned in more depth in the next chapter). The trauma that was experienced by soldiers seemed to respond well with talk therapy, therefore, a new classification scheme called the *Medical 203* was conceived and reflected conditions that were psychological as opposed to biological and congenital. The conditions of war, especially those which produced war trauma prompted this document, which was commissioned by the Surgeon General and supported by the U.S. Military (Clegg, 2012).

Since the soldiers reacted well to the talk therapy during World War II, the psychotherapeutic approach was maintained by psychiatrists afterward, even as the mentally ill patients began to be treated in the community instead of mental hospitals. During the war, many physicians with specialties other than psychiatry decided to work in mental health, causing the number of psychiatrists in the post-war period to swell rapidly. A group of young psychiatrists calling themselves the Young Turks began to organize within the American Psychiatric Association and sought to focus more on the social problems associated with mental illness. And, they sought to create a new classification system, one that reflected the new focus on psychotherapy (particularly psychoanalysis) and a broader approach to mental health provision.

The DSM and its Progeny

The original DSM (here called DSM-I to distinguish it from the later versions) had a panel of mental health experts who provided their opinions on the symptoms that made up a specific "mental disease"—the most "yes" votes determined the new diagnostic label (Concalves et al., 2002). The DSM-1 was considered by some to be an extension of the *Statistical Manual*, though others claim it was more like the *Medical 203* because much of its terminology was the same and the psychoanalytic approach was maintained (Clegg, 2012). In 1950, a draft of the new manual with the new nosology was circulated to mental health organizations and presented to the American Psychiatric Association (APA) (Grob, 1991). The manual, which has gone through several versions, was first published in 1952 by the APA to firm up a loosely governed process of diagnosis of the mental health needs of soldiers during and after the Second World War (Malik & Beutler, 2002; Clegg, 2012).

The DSM-II was produced many years later, in 1968, and attempted to align more closely with the highly influential ICD (International Classification of Diseases, produced by the World Health Organization, or WHO) (Clegg, 2012), the other primary classification document in the mental health field. The DSM-II adopted some new diagnostic names, descriptions, and classifications with a new section on disorders associated with childhood (Clegg, 2012). The 1960s and 1970s saw a major change in the mental health field, most notably psychiatry. A growing cause commonly labeled the "anti-psychiatry movement" began and was promoted by psychiatrists Thomas Szasz and R.D. Laing and sociologists Thomas Scheff and Erving Goffman, among other practitioners and scholars. The anti-psychiatrists saw the label of mental illness promoted by the DSM as being of questionable merit, more appropriately interpreted as an indication of other social processes, and even detrimental to mental health clients as well as the mental health system.

In 1980, the DSM-III was published. It reflected a major change from the first two editions in that it was much larger, more comprehensive, and represented a shift in the mental health field by eschewing the psychological perspective of the first two editions on mental disorders and returning to a bio-medical approach, resurrecting the earlier model espoused by

Kraepelin (Kirk & Kutchins, 1992). It sought to clearly differentiate normal from abnormal using empirical evidence to make it (at least appear to be) a scientific manual (Frances, 2013). It discarded the theoretical basis (primarily that of psychoanalysis) of the first two editions and focused more on empirical data to form clusters to create the diagnostic categories (Clegg, 2012). The DSM-III was designed not only to create a scientific, standardized nosology, but it was also forged from the pressure from the insurance industry who demanded reliable diagnoses, treatment methods, and predictable outcomes; psychiatry changed to accommodate this demand. In addition to the insurance companies' influence on the manual, the growth of the personal computer, which quickly crunches numbers and provides quantifiable data for research and diagnostic examinations (in the process removing human intuition and running the risk of turning treatment providers into "caretakers of machines") also prompted the changes in the third edition (LaBruzza, 1997).

In 1987, a revision to the DSM-III, the DSM-III-R (the "R" stands for revision) was published to add recommendations from the team working on the ICD-10 and to correct some diagnostic criteria in the previous edition that seemed to conflict with the results of new studies. Categories were renamed and reorganized, and new ones were added (most notably the category "developmental disorders") and some diagnostic criteria were changed for some illnesses (Clegg, 2012). The DSM-III is especially notable as it removed the classification of homosexuality as a mental disorder, after much protest from gay activists after the release of the DSM II (in the seventh revision of the DSM II it was changed to Sexual Orientation Disturbance). However, it was replaced in the DSM III with something called Ego-Dystonic Homosexuality which was meant for patients who were having psychological complications due to their sexual orientation. When the DSM-III-R was released, Ego-Dystonic Homosexuality was removed, signaling an end to the hotly debated homosexuality-as-mental disorder argument (Kirk & Kutchins, 1992). And although sleep disorders were mentioned in the DSM II and DSM III as conditions affecting the mental functioning of people, particularly children, the DSM-III-R officially made sleep disorders a mental illness (Houts, 2002), a change that has continued to the most recent edition, which lists over two dozen "sleep-wake" disorders in more than 60 pages of text.

The American Psychiatric Association released the DSM-IV in 1994, which continued its coordination with the newest edition of the ICD of that time, the ICD-10. The new DSM reorganized categories from the previous edition but had no major changes in its theoretical underpinnings. It did include an interesting addition in terms of "culture" by taking cultural variation into account when performing mental health diagnoses (Clegg, 2012); this is possibly a reflection of societal changes that took a more multicultural and inclusive approach during the period. The DSM-IV-TR (text revision) was published in 2000, and while it incorporated some diagnostic criteria in a few areas and provided updated information, it reflected few major changes from the DSM-IV, including changes in diagnostic categories (Clegg, 2012). The axial system (later dropped in the DSM-5) consisted of disorders in 5 categories:

- Axis I consisted of mental disorders such as mood disorders, psychotic disorders, eating disorders, dissociative disorders, and substance-related disorders
- Axis II was comprised of the personality disorders and developmental disorders
- Axis III disorders were conditions related to physical problems
- Axis IV consisted of social and environmental disorders
- Axis IV was a so-called Global Assessment of Functioning Scale which provided a quantitative scale to assess daily living functioning.

THE ASSESSMENT OF SUBSTANCE-RELATED AND ADDICTIVE DISORDERS

Prior to its entrance in the DSM, substance abuse assessment and classification depended on rudimentary nosological schemes developed in the 20th century. In 1937, a system was developed and offered but two categories—symptomatic drinking, which was alcoholism that developed as an attempt to mask underlying mental and physical conditions, and true alcohol addiction which contained the symptoms of dependence and withdrawal, and which was believed to be a distinct clinical disorder. In 1942, famed addiction researcher and Yale professor E.M. Jelinek, created a classification scheme which involved fourteen categories on a continuum from "exuberant drinker" and "occupational drinker" to "decadent drinker" and "true addict". In 1960, he developed a new system with five categories of alcoholism based on the Greek alphabet:

1. Alpha type—addiction with psychological dependence
2. Beta type—physical problems related to alcohol use but without physical or psychological dependence
3. Gamma type—a severe condition with psychological dependence progressing to physical dependence
4. Delta type—heavy drinking leading to physical addiction

5. Epsilon type—a condition defined by binge drinking followed by periods of abstinence (White, 2014).

In 1952 substance use was included in the DSM-I as acute and chronic brain syndromes (due to alcohol, other drugs, and poison), listed as personality disorders in the form of addiction, alcoholism, and drug addiction and in a category called alcoholic intoxication (simple drunkenness). In the DSM-II, substance use was simply labeled as alcoholism and drug dependence and included a few specifiers. As noted before, the DSM-III heralded a less theoretical and more scientific framework and in the DSM IV-TR, substance-use disorders ended up primarily in the category of Axis I disorders.

Describing a need for a new classification for addiction, Fatayer (2008) suggests a new diagnostic typology:

1. Alpha addiction that includes addiction to foods
2. Beta addiction that includes chemical substances
3. Gamma addiction that consists of behavioral addictions
4. Delta addiction that consists of a combination of at least two of the other types (in which there is a distinction between primary and secondary addictions)

This new proposed classification is intended for several reasons, including enhancing diagnosis of substance and behavioral disorders, promoting a better plan of treatment, and minimizing the stigma associated with addiction.

The DSM-5, the Current Edition

The most current DSM is markedly different than its predecessors in many ways. Perhaps the most obvious is that the DSM-5 is designated by a number rather than a Roman Numeral (unlike DSM-II, DSM-III, and DSM-IV); this is to make an easier transition to an online format, as the next editions will probably be DSM-5.2 and so on (Lieberman, 2015).

As with its predecessors, each mental disorder has a detailed description of the problem and has the following sections:

- *Diagnostic Criteria and Descriptors,* like its predecessors, presents in abbreviated table and text formats complete with information and numerical code (for example, Antisocial Personality Disorder in the DSM-5 is 301.7)

- *Associated Features Supporting Diagnosis* (which provides more information such as in Panic Disorder, coded as 300.01), where there is information about "an unexpected type of panic attack is a nocturnal panic attack" (American Psychiatric Association, 2013, p. 210)
- The *Prevalence* section explains how common the disorder is in the general or special population, based on research data. An example is that for Kleptomania, 312.32, the disorder occurs "in about 4-24% of individuals arrested for shoplifting. Its prevalence in the general population is very rare, at approximately 0.3-0.6%. Females outnumber males at a ratio of 3:1" (APA, 2013, p. 478).
- A section called *Development and Course* provides information about how the disorder normally appears and develops, for example, Dissociative Amnesia, 300.12, has this feature: "onset of generalized amnesia is usually sudden" (APA, 2013, p. 299).
- *Subtypes* and *Specifiers* which are mentioned in some disorders further supports diagnostic information, for example, a subtype of Anorexia Nervosa, 307.1, is the "binge-eating/purging type" (APA, 2013, p. 339), and a specifier for Hoarding Disorder, 300.3, requires the diagnostician to specify if the disorder is "with excessive acquisition" (APA, 2013, p. 248)
- *Risk and Prognostic Features* section gives different types of risk situations (temperament, environmental, genetic/physiological) that affect prognosis (APA, 2013)
- The *Differential Diagnosis* section provides information for ruling out other potential diagnoses (APA, 2013).

There is more information given on the illnesses in the DSM-5 in sections called *Medication-induced Movement Disorders and other Conditions that May be a Focus of Clinical Attention, Culture-Related Diagnostic Issues, Gender-Related Diagnostic Issues, Functional Consequences, Suicide Risk,* and *Comorbidity.* And there are a host "other" and "unspecified" categories that seek to narrow the description of the condition. Again, different disorders in the guide have different sections, however, all will have some or most of these. Therefore, there is much diagnostic information in the highly detailed DSM-5.

There are many structural and organizational changes in the current DSM and it goes well beyond the scope of this book to list them all. However, a few of the controversial ones will be discussed. In the section on trauma, posttraumatic stress has been moved from the anxiety disorder section to a separate section along with other disorders that seems to reject the salient issue of anxiety in these conditions. In the autism disorder section, Asperger's Syndrome, which has some notable differences with other conditions related to other forms of autism, was removed and disorders with similar features were placed on a spectrum, or continuum, of disorders. Another controversy is the diagnosis of depression, which after a few days of grief, can now be considered a mental disorder. An additional controversial diagnosis has been made for young people who might be at risk for psychosis later in life—Attenuated Psychoses Syndrome, or Psychotic Risk Syndrome, which appears in the *Conditions for Further Study* section (which means the syndrome is not officially a clinical diagnosis at this time but one with potential for inclusion in a subsequent DSM) provides that a person with a potential for psychosis may be so diagnosed to prevent a full-blown psychotic condition; perhaps well intended, this has the consequence of labeling someone, perhaps mistakenly, that will create a self-fulfilling prophecy that allows the symptomology to be maintained. These are but a few of the concerns regarding the most recent DSM.

It is interesting to observe the progression of the DSM series. The original DSM had 106 diagnoses and had 128 pages while the DSM-II had only 6 more diagnoses than the original (134) but the number of pages increased to 182. The DSM-III evidenced much growth and adopted a full book format rather than the small, spiral-bound versions of its predecessors; it totaled 265 diagnoses and increased to 494 pages and its revision jumped to 292 diagnoses and 567 pages. The DSM-IV continued to grow to 365 diagnoses and a whopping 888 pages (Malik & Beutler, 2002). By the time the DSM-IV-TR hit the market, it had 943 pages. The growth has certainly continued as the DSM-5 has 947 pages (it is difficult to confirm the exact number of disorders due to the convoluted nature of categorization). This might suggest the increase is due to a better categorization of disorders with much better empirical support or it might suggest that too many common living problems are now becoming medicalized. We will explore this further in subsequent chapters.

It will be interesting to see how mental disorders will be diagnosed in the future, since our diagnostic categorization can tell us much about the way mental health is perceived and what cultural and environmental factors guide these decisions. It also creates many questions including:

- Will the DSM still be the prominent diagnostic guide?
- If so, will it continue to grow and add more diagnoses?
- If so, will the manual be strictly offered online due to its cumbersome size?

- Additionally, does this inclusion of so many conditions signal the overmedicalization of normal aspects of living and expose the source of diagnostic inflation?
- And who benefits from this "diagnostic inflation" (Frances, 2013)—Big Pharma, the medical field generally?

It could be that diagnostic inflation contributes to a much larger field of disorders, therefore promoting the growth of what has been termed the "mental health enterprise" (Kirk & Kutchins, 1992, p. 8). If there is a large field of disorders and an ambiguous characterization of these disorders, misdiagnosis could naturally occur. (For a good discussion on concerns of misdiagnosis, see Frances, 2013).

Some practitioners and scholars are pleased with the DSM, arguing that such a classification must exist to effectively diagnose and treat mental disorders because standards must be derived for diagnosis (and treatment) to be effective and scientifically-based. And, of course, there are financial concerns—insurance providers demand a degree of accountability that is an outcome of a consistent diagnostic system. However, a group of psychiatrists strongly opposed to the DSM, particularly the most recent incarnation (mirroring the 1960s and 1970s anti-psychiatrists mentioned earlier), are concerned that "toxic psychiatry" (Breggin, 1994) is taking over the field of mental health diagnosis through over-medicalization—medicalizing behaviors that are part of human existence (or what Thomas Szasz called "problems in living")—that can hardly be considered mental problems. We can look at conditions such as Sleep Apnea: this is a medical problem that causes distress, but is it a mental problem in itself? How about Social Phobia—is it a mental illness to be shy in social situations? Another issue involves behaviors that have been classified as mental disorders such as Pyromania and Kleptomania—are these mental problems or, more appropriately, the crimes of arson and theft?

Some scholars and practitioners have pondered the possibility of an alternative to the DSM. Sheltered under the protective umbrella of the medical profession, it likely will be difficult for some alternate diagnostic guide, perhaps one that is more qualitative in nature, to successfully emerge. Mental health diagnoses are closely tied to treatments, including psychopharmacology, therefore, something short of a highly scientific guide would probably prove less medically and legally sound. And of course, these mental health diagnoses are tied to forensic determinations in the determination of court sentences or commitment to mental institutions. A recent, novel approach is provided by historian Edward Shorter (Shorter, 2015). His "alternative nosology", which he admits does not include all currently accepted disorders, consists of a return to the pre-DSM period by erasing the distinctions between mood disorders and psychosis, and those of depression and anxiety, and by returning to the classic delineation between psychosis and neurosis (for more information on this proposed classification system, see Shorter, 2015).

The DSM is a product of the American Psychiatric Association and, hate it or love it, is the predominant diagnostic manual in the field, rivaled in use only by the ICD series, which is coupled with the DSM. Since the DSM is a creation of American psychiatry, it is often viewed with skepticism by some of the other mental health workers who also provide mental health diagnoses. We will take up this matter in our section on "the psy-professionals". The DSM series is more than just an evolving classification of mental disorders; it represents cultural shifts and the grappling by society with mental health problems. And it reflects the changing field of psychiatry that has taken upon itself the issue of diagnosis.

A sound mental health classification and diagnostic program is integral to the mental health system. If there are potential alternatives to the current system (such as those proposed by Fatayer and Shorter in this chapter), these might be useful, at least to start a conversation. It is possible that other sectors of the mental health establishment (such as clinical or counseling psychology, clinical social work, or marriage and family therapy) might have input into upcoming nosologies. Or it might be that academic disciplines, such as sociology or psychology, provide input in the process. It is also possible that advocacy groups external to clinical practice or academia—groups that represent patients and their families—might also be a resource for classification changes. In any event, observing the course of mental health diagnosis provides a rich sociological understanding of mental health and how society deals with deviations from normative mental health behavior.

Now we will turn to the mental health disorders and we will use the DSM-5 (APA, 2013) to guide us through the disorders due to its preeminence in the field of mental health. We will examine the disorders of mental health generally then follow the structure of the DSM-5 to examine the specific disorders listed therein, starting with the those at the beginning of the guide, then following along accordingly, describing all the disorders, including those that are in the manual but that have not been considered "madness" at earlier times. Please note that the descriptions are a brief synopsis of some of the disorders in the designated categories and exclude detailed information, subsections, specifiers, etc.; refer to the DSM-5 to get specific details of the disorders.

MENTAL DISORDERS

Mental disorders come in a wide range of types. Some have a biological basis while others are more likely to be caused by, or least exacerbated by, stressors in the social environment. And many likely have a combination of both. Some can be treated by medications while others are unaffected by them, or have their conditions worsened by their use. Some fall distinctly in the mental disorder category while others are questionable and could be better characterized as physical disorders, or emotional manifestations of physical problems. All fall along a spectrum of severity and the level of anguish caused by the condition. Many appear to overlap, and many people suffer from more than one disorder. All involve, to varying degrees, a loss of control. And all of them can benefit from professional help. The DSM-5 provides these conditions as mental disorders:

Neurodevelopmental Disorders—these are the disorders that usually manifest in childhood that have a neurological cause and that continue through the life span. Included in this large category are Intellectual Disabilities (previously referred to as Developmental Disorders), Communication Disorders, Autism Spectrum Disorder, Attention-Deficit/Hyperactivity Disorder (ADHD), Specific Learning Disorder, and Motor Disorders.

Schizophrenia Spectrum and other Psychotic Disorders—these are the disorders with psychotic features and involve delusions, hallucinations (visual, audial, or other sensory modality) disordered thinking, and disorganized motor activity. Disorders such as Schizophrenia, Schizotypal Disorder, Schizoaffective Disorder, Catatonia, and Delusional Disorder are part of this spectrum. Note—the idea of a spectrum suggests a continuum of characteristics and related symptomology.

Bipolar and Related Disorders—bipolar disorder (previously referred to as Manic-Depressive Disorder to describe the alternating pattern of mania and depression) is represented in Bipolar I and Bipolar II, and Cyclothymic Disorder. In manic phases, people in these categories experience elevated mood, increased activity, euphoria, irritability, and flight of ideas; when in the depressed phase, people experience depressed mood, sadness, decreased energy, and feelings of hopelessness.

Depressive Disorders—these are the mood disorders that represent sadness, emptiness, irritability, anhedonia (the inability to experience pleasure), and the physical and cognitive responses that are connected to these conditions. Included in this group are Major Depressive Disorder, Persistent Depressive Disorder (previously called Dysthymia), and Premenstrual Dysphoric Disorder; these disorders are separated by the duration of the illnesses, along with timing and their presumed causes.

Anxiety Disorders—the disorders in this category include Separation Anxiety Disorder, Specific Phobia, Social Anxiety Disorder (previously called Social Phobia), Panic Disorder, Agoraphobia, and General Anxiety Disorder. All anxiety disorders have at their core disturbances resulting from fear and anxiety—fear refers to a reaction to a real or imagined threat while anxiety refers to the anticipation of such a threat.

Obsessive-Compulsive and Related Disorders—refer to disorders in which the sufferer has obsessions (thoughts or urges that are persistent and troubling that a person consistently ponders) and compulsions (behaviors that are insistently performed to relieve the obsessive thought patterns). Included in this category are Obsessive-Compulsive Disorder (often referred to by its initials, OCD), Body Dysmorphic Disorder, Trichotillomania (hair pulling), Excoriation (skin-picking), and the newly added Hoarding Disorder.

Trauma- and Stressor-Related Disorders—these disorders are related to the experience of a real or perceived threat creates stress and anxiety. They include Post-Traumatic Stress Disorder, Reactive Attachment Disorder, Reactive Attachment Disorder, Disinhibited Stress Engagement Disorder, Acute Stress Disorder, and Adjustment Disorders.

Dissociative Disorders—dissociative disorders are those in which people have a disruption in consciousness, perception, body representation, and memory. People with these illnesses may feel unconnected with reality, with themselves, with their surroundings, or with their pasts (in the form of amnesia). Examples are Dissociative Identity Disorder, Dissociative Amnesia, and Depersonalization/Derealization Disorder.

Somatic Symptom and Related Disorders—these are emotional disorders that reflect physical conditions in which the people suffering from them are primarily seen in medical settings such as primary care institutions rather than mental health establishments. Examples include Somatic Symptom Disorder, Illness Anxiety Disorder, and Conversion Disorder.

Feeding and Eating Disorders—the disorders in this category all involve the emotional and psychological disturbances involved in the process of consuming food. Examples are Anorexia Nervosa, Bulimia Nervosa, Binge-Eating Disorder, Rumination Disorder, Avoidant/Restrictive Intake Disorder and Pica (which involves eating non-food items).

Elimination Disorders—these disorders include behaviors that involve the elimination of urine and fecal matter from the body in inappropriate ways and places. Often first manifested in childhood and adolescence, examples are Enuresis (the elimination of urine from the body) and Encopresis (the elimination of feces).

Sleep-Wake Disorders—this is a lengthy section that in many ways reflects the ways in which inappropriate sleep patterns (involving quality, timing, and amount of sleep) can cause psychological issues. These conditions include Insomnia Disorder, Narcolepsy, Obstructive Sleep Apnea, Sleep-Related Hypoventilation, and Circadian Rhythm Sleep-Wake Disorders.

Sexual Dysfunctions—this section includes problems in sexual activity and, as in the last section, deals with the psychological effect of conditions that inhibit a person's ability to respond to or enjoy sexuality; included are Delayed Ejaculation, Erectile Disorder, and Female Orgasmic Disorder.

Gender Dysphoria—this section is dedicated exclusively to gender dysphoria and includes Gender Dysphoria and Other Specified- and Unspecified Gender Dysphoria. This condition addresses controversial transgender issues and refers to the discomfort and distress experienced by people who experience an incongruence between their expressed and assigned gender, especially if reassignment measures are unavailable. The term gender dysphoria replaces the DSM-IV's use of Gender Identity Disorder to note the problematic condition is the clinical issue rather than a person's identity.

Disruptive, Impulse-Control, and Conduct Disorders—these disorders involve impulse control behaviors, such as aggression and violence, that result in the violation of the rights of others. Examples are Oppositional Defiant Disorder, Intermittent Explosive Disorder, Conduct Disorder), Antisocial Personality Disorder, Pyromania (fire-setting), and Kleptomania (theft). These disorders often involve the criminal justice system due to their close connection with injury to others (physical or psychological), destruction of property, or other forms of behavior deemed criminal.

Substance-Related and Addictive Disorders—this section explains key terms in the diagnosis and clinical treatment of substance use and addictive disorders. This category covers 10 substance abuse disorders based on these drug classes: alcohol; caffeine; cannabis; hallucinogens; inhalants; opioids; sedatives, hypnotics and anxiolytics; stimulants; tobacco; and other or unknown drugs. The DSM-5 has added a special class of addiction—Non-Substance Related Disorder, which refers to behavioral addiction. Gambling is the activity that received the nod to be the first behavioral addiction in the guide. The DSM-5 hints that Internet Gaming might be classified as a behavioral addiction in the future if the empirical research suggests it is relevant; the manual also mentions other potential behavioral addictions—sex addiction, exercise addiction, and shopping addiction, however, the research has not currently established the evidence for these behaviors. This is an unusually large section in the DSM-5 and constitutes over 100 pages (compare this to the previous section on Disruptive, Impulse-Control and Conduct Disorders which has 20 pages or the section on Gender Dysphoria, which has 9 pages).

Neurocognitive Disorders—this section refers to disorders involving cognitive functioning due to biomedical causes. Included are Delirium and a long list of Major or Mild Neurocognitive Disorders (resulting from Alzheimer's Disease, Lewy Bodies, Vascular Disease, HIV infection, Prion Disease, Parkinson's Disease, Huntington's Disease, or other medical conditions).

Personality Disorders—the group of disorders known as personality disorders are characterized by personality traits that are inflexible and maladaptive and that generate behaviors that deviate sharply from the person's cultural norms. There are many disorders in this grouping that have varying characteristics, manifestations, and symptoms. Included in this category are Antisocial Personality Disorder, Borderline Personality Disorder, Narcissistic Personality Disorder, Histrionic Personality Disorder, and Schizoid Personality Disorder. Antisocial Personality Disorder, often used by its non-clinical name, sociopathy or psychopathy, is notable in that it involves a mental orientation involving criminality.

Paraphilic Disorders—these disorders involve sexual behavior often considered deviant that contain harmful or potentially harmful consequences to others. Included are Voyeuristic Disorder, Exhibitionistic Disorder, Frotteuristic Disorder, Sexual Masochism Disorder, Sexual Sadism Disorder, Pedophilic Disorder, and Fetishistic Disorder. These disorders are closely tied with the criminal justice system as others are often harmed in the commission of paraphilic behaviors.

Other Mental Disorders, Medication-Induced Movement Disorders, Other Adverse Effects of Medication, and *Other Conditions That May Be a Focus of Clinical Attention*—these are the last categories that round out all the disorders not previously covered. The last section contains the *V codes* that are specifically addressed as not being mental orders but circumstances that might affect patients seen in practice: these include relational problems (with significant others), abuse and neglect, and a host of other personal and environmental circumstances that affect a person's mental well-being.

THE PSY-PROFESSIONALS

There are many different types of professional psychotherapists whose function is to work with people with mental and emotional issues. Some work as private therapists, others work at mental health clinics, and others work at mental health facilities. They have different types and levels of education, training, and different treatment emphases. They often use different training modalities and disciple-specific ways of "doing therapy". Some work primarily in individual therapy, others in group therapy, some do co-therapy, and many do a combination of these methods, depending on the circumstances. All "psy-professionals" (Cohen, 2016) work with individuals, groups, families, however, regardless of their professional orientation. All have their own governing professional organizations that provide guidance and codes of conduct. And they all use the most current DSM for diagnostic and treatment guidance. But they are all mental health practitioners, and all seek to alleviate the problems of people having emotional difficulties.

Psychiatrists

Many of us are familiar with the position of psychiatrist and some people automatically think of this position when they think of mental health professions. Psychiatrists are licensed medical doctors and are often considered the "top of the food chain" in the mental health enterprise. Psychiatrists must have an M.D., followed by a four-year residency in a psychiatric setting, and two or more years in a specialty area. The activities of psychiatrists are governed by the American Psychiatric Association (APA), their primary professional organization, an organization of 37,000 members (APA, n.d.). The American Medical Association (AMA) is the principle professional association for medical doctors of all specializations. As noted before, the psychiatrists took on the oversight of the DSM diagnostic classification systems.

Psychologists

Another well-known group of mental health practitioners are the psychologists. Psychologists are nonmedical practitioners and typically have a Ph.D. (Doctor of Philosophy) in psychology; some psychologists have what is known as a Psy.D. (Doctor of Psychology), a degree of that focuses more on applied clinical work than the Ph.D., or an Ed.D. (Doctor of Education). Some psychologists who work in certain environments, such as state or federal institutions, research organizations, and institutions of higher education are exempt from the doctoral requirement. Psychologists must perform a 2,000-hour clinical internship and a 2,000-postdoctoral program, though school psychologists might have other requirements as deemed appropriate by that state's department of education. Psychologists are primarily interested in mental health diagnosis and treatment and, like the other non-medical therapists, do not normally prescribe or monitor medications. There are many subfields in psychology such as clinical psychology, counseling psychology, community psychology, developmental psychology, industrial/organizational (I/O) psychology, school psychology, and social psychology. The primary professional association for psychologists is the American Psychological Association (the "other APA") which has over 115,700 members (APA, n.d.). Since psychologists take less of a medical approach to diagnosis and treatment than psychiatrists, they sometimes have issues with diagnostic principles, certainly since the DSM III came into existence, and scholars believe psychology has some alternatives to the strict medical nosology of the diagnostic guide (see Pilgrim, 2014).

Social Workers

Social workers constitute a large group of psy-professionals. Social workers normally have at least a master's degree in Social Work (MSW), though some have a Ph.D. in Social Work or a DSW (Doctor of Social Work). In some states, a Bachelor of Social Work (BSW) degree will allow someone to obtain licensure and practice psychotherapy. Social work practitioners achieve licensure as a Licensed Clinical Social Worker (LCSW), Licensed Independent Social Worker (LISW) or Licensed Independent Clinical Social Worker (LICSW), depending on the name granted by the state. LCSWs require 2 years of documented clinical supervision post degree, a passing score on a national exam for social workers and completion of CEUs to maintain licensure. The professional organization that oversees social work practice is the National Association of Social Workers (NASW), an old organization currently maintaining over 100,000 members (NASW, n.d.). Social work practitioners focus primarily on assisting *clients* (rather than *patients*, redirecting attention from the medical model to a psychosocial one) with an understanding of service and resource utilization from a variety of areas. Like psychologists, there is sometimes an uneasy relationship with the DSM and, especially due to their social work orientation, many social workers express concern that a strictly medical strategy of diagnosis and treatment ignores important social, economic, and cultural issues that can impede individual mental wellbeing (Robbins, 2014). A "psychological justice" approach is often adopted in which clients are taught psychosocial skills that provide a complement to the environment they inhabit (Wakefield, 2013).

Marriage and Family Therapists

Marriage and family therapists (MFTs) have completed at least a master's degree with a family-focused curriculum, though some have a Ph.D. They also must complete a 2-year post-master's clinical supervision program, pass a national exam in family therapy, and they must maintain their license through the acquisition of CEUs. Their focus is on how mental problems and relational problems are found (and maintained) in former and current family patterns of interaction, that is, they take a "systems" view of mental problems. MFTs do not normally distinguish an identified single patient as all members of the family are viewed as the patient. The organization that provides supervision to this group is the American Association of Marriage and Family Therapists (AAMFT) and the national agency has affiliations in all states with over 25,000 members. Practitioners in family therapy have experienced a 50 fold increase in their numbers since 1970 and there are now over 50,000 MFTs in the U.S. (AAMFT, n.d.) There has always existed a natural disinclination with this group to adhere to the DSM diagnosis due to the manual's focus on medicalizing mental disorder in lieu of observing the rich range of human experiences and relationships so desired by MFTs; the response to the DSM-5, then, has not been a warm one (Larner, Strong, & Busch, 2013).

Mental Health Counselors

Mental health counselors also constitute a large part of the mental health practitioner field. They are licensed in some states as License Professional Counselors (LPCs), or in other states as Licensed Mental Health Counselors (LMHC) or Licensed Clinical Counselors (LCCs). A master's degree in psychology or another counseling discipline, 3,000 hours of clinical supervision over 2 years, and a passing score on a national mental health counselor exam are required for licensure. Some practitioners also have a doctoral degree in the field. The nation's LPCs, numbering around 120,000, are primarily governed by the American Counseling Association (ACA), boasting a membership of 55,000 (ACA, n.d.). LMHCs formulate diagnoses and provide treatment, and, like the other psy-professionals, rely on the DSM for their guidance in these areas. Counseling scholars suggest the strong neurological and biological emphasis of the DSM fails to address psychological and social variables and suggest ways to reframe diagnosis to included multicultural and social justice perspectives (See Zalaquett, Fuerth, Stein, Ivey, & Bradford Ivey 2008).

Psychiatric Nurses

Psychiatric-mental health nurses (PMHNs) are medical mental health providers who develop a nursing plan of treatment, provide nursing care, and formulate a treatment evaluation. Psychiatric-mental health advance practice registered nurses (PMH-APRNs) have master's or doctoral degrees and assess, diagnose, prescribe medications, and provide nursing care to people with mental health needs. PMHNs must have at least an RN license, 2 years of primary nursing experience, and 2,000 hours of mental health nursing. The largest professional organization for PMHNs is the American Psychiatric Nurses Association which boasts a membership of over 10,000 nurses (APNA, n.d.). These providers are closely tied to psychiatry and do much of the same therapeutic work of psychiatrists, especially the advance practice nurses, however, some psychiatric nurses acknowledge feelings of disregard as they are relegated to using the DSM, but having limited contributions as new editions are being produced (Pearson, 2013).

CONCLUSION

The assessment of mental disorders is the beginning stage of an effective treatment program. There is a long history of diagnosis in the mental health field which has culminated in the Diagnostic and Statistical Manual of Mental Disorders (DSM) and its revisions. The evolution of the DSM provides insight as to how the mental health system (and the greater society) views the assessment of mental disorders. The increase in the number of conditions considered to be mental disorders continues to grow dramatically in the continuing revisions of the manual. Concerns of the medicalization of normal life problems has been suggested by many scholars and practitioners, however, many see the inclusion of these conditions as creating a more functional system, reaching larger numbers of people.

The psychiatric view of mental disorders is based on the medical model. An examination is made, and a course of treatment is prepared, often involving pharmacological interventions. The sociological view has a different perspective and questions the legitimacy of the classification of mental disorders, which are perceived as labels whose consequences create more problems for those so labeled. The anti-psychiatrists of the 1960s and 1970s sought to draw attention to this labeling process and to redefine the disorders, at least some of them, as "problems in living", eschewing the clinical labeling process as well as the use of the medical model. Currently, there are other groups of scholars and practitioners who view the current diagnosis and treatment processes as being "toxic", or detrimental, and who rail against not only the diagnostic process but also psychopharmacological approaches. However, a standardized system of assessment is required in a complex society and if the current classification system is deemed ineffective, other alternative nosologies might appear on the scene.

There are many practitioners in the mental health field. The top tier of this stratified system is claimed by psychiatrists, medical doctors who specialize in treating mental disorders. Psychologists are primarily doctoral level non-medical therapists who treat a broad variety of disorders and have traditionally had assessment as a focal point of their practice. Social workers have a long history in the mental health field and emphasize social aspects of client's lives and seek support systems in the community. Marriage and family therapists see the entire family as the patient and look to the family for both the origin of dysfunctions in a person's life and the potential for positive change. Mental health counselors often have a background in counseling psychology and provide an array of counseling services to clients. Psychiatric nurses are mental health practitioners who normally work in medical settings and have the ability, as nurses, to offer a variety of clinical services.

Sometimes it appears that the current mental health scheme that we currently follow is the only possible outgrowth of the application of mental health services. There are, of course, many other possibilities—we have seen the historical contexts of understandings and treatment of the mentally ill. Underlying the classification of certain behaviors and the practitioners that have been given the mandate to "heal" are the cultural values and beliefs that drive our assumptions on how to diagnose and treat those behaviors. The therapeutic substructure exposes our ideals that rely on observation (that certain behaviors constitute mental illness) as well as the use of scientific data upon which to make diagnoses that are valid, and treatment protocols that conform to best practices and that are evidence based. Science and rationalization are the basic drivers of diagnosis and the formal processes involving certifying our practitioners to do the important work of psychotherapy.

Chapter 4

CURRENT PSYCHOTHERAPY APPROACHES

"And then, how do I describe the play, the creative process by which I become audience and participant, leader of the therapy and also a member of the therapeutic system, and the by-ways that family members follow while they experience new, better ways of relating?" (Salvador Minuchin, Wai-Yung Lee, and George M. Simon 1996, p. 58)

MENTAL HEALTH AND SUBSTANCE ABUSE TREATMENT

The treatment measures in this chapter will begin with some older methods we now find appalling, but it is important to review them, certainly not for their quaintness but to illustrate the progression of our understandings of both mental illness and its treatment. Mental health and substance abuse treatments are separated in this chapter due to some differences that have existed in our understandings of the two, however, since many treatments apply to both, these commonalities will be noted.

It could be said that psychotherapy's roots could be found in the work of the shaman and healers of ancient times and it is true there are some similarities. These predecessors sought to use magic and later spirituality to help troubled souls, but as modernity arrived many changes required the establishment of a professional discipline. As noted in the last chapter, psychiatry developed within the already established field of medicine and later other fields were created or adapted to take on the task of providing psychotherapy. As with other chapters, we will begin with a brief history of mental health treatment, to help review the roadmap that has developed to the practice we now know as psychotherapy.

Early mental illness "treatments"

Some of the earliest "treatments" that were used for mental illness we would find shocking today. For example, trephination (the drilling of holes in the skull) was commonly used among the ancients to allow the demons thought to cause the disturbances to escape from the mind; skulls found by archaeologists attest to this early treatment that was practiced in many parts of the world until the middle ages (Hajar, 2012). The ancient Greeks, concerned that madness was a sign of demonic possession, sang, spoke, and chanted words and gibberish, often accompanied by a lyre, to convince the unwelcome visitor (by fright, deception, or persuasion) to leave the possessed. It would seem as if the treatment was focused on the demons rather than the people suffering from madness. Later, these poor folks were beaten, almost drowned, and frightened to get the devils to find another home—unfortunately, they could simply find any other human body to take up residence. This practice continued through the eighteenth century but virtually disappeared by the nineteenth century (Altschule, 1977). Certainly, the "treatment" as practiced here seems more closely aligned to exorcism.

Later, amulets, charms, and holy relics were used in Europe to allay madness, objects which were later replaced with magnets. Magnetism was based on the idea that the body has magnetic properties and when the internal magnets became weakened, external magnets were applied to the body to retain balance. Some have heard the term "animal magnetism" but have ideas different than the way it was intended. Anton Mesmer (of mesmerism fame) believed that the planets influenced human behavior due to a special fluid called animal magnetism, which produced a group of healers known as "animal magnetizers" or "mesmerists", who used a large variety of devices to restore appropriate levels of magnetism (Altschule, 1977). Mesmerism would later evolve into hypnotism which was later adopted by Sigmund Freud until he found it ineffective in treating patients; he later turned to other methods to uncover the root of some of the problems of his patients who suffered from neurosis.

Treatments that utilized fear and shock have a very long history and have been manifest in many methods. The "surprise bath" consisted of immersing the mad into water or throwing them into it (Altschule, 1977). Another form of shock therapy involving water was the use of a chair to dunk people into frigid water, with the hope that the intimidation factor would alleviate the problem (Zwelling, 1985). However, water was not always used to shock patients—sedative baths were humane and soothing and recommended by many early physicians (Altschule, 1977).

Chairs with straps were commonly used to restrain patients before the fabled straitjacket was used for this purpose. Benjamin Rush created the "tranquilizer", a chair into which the patient was strapped; this device had a specific box that was placed over the patient's head to allow complete quiet. Sometimes cold water was placed on top of the box to cool the fevers of the mind. Interestingly, even this was more humane than some of the contraptions used in Europe at the time, such as dunking cages and swinging chairs that were used to force the mad to sanity (Scull, 2015). Those considered mad were bled, blistered, made to vomit and sweat, and frightened—certainly not acceptable forms of treatment today.

As mentioned earlier, at the turn of the twentieth century, those deemed "morally defective" were subjected to involuntary sterilization to stop them from producing more of their kind. The mentally ill were severely looked down even more than the other pariahs of the day: immigrants, criminal offenders, and racial minorities. They were viewed as primitive barbarians and were sterilized until the practice eventually resulted in public notice and scorn (Whitaker, 2002).

In the early 1920s, barbiturates were given to the mentally ill to induce long periods of sleep. In the next decade, insulin and a drug called Metrazol were used to induce seizures in schizophrenics with the intention of shocking the body violently enough to remove the madness from the person's mind. By the decade's end, electricity was used (termed electroconvulsive therapy or ECT). Psychosurgery, in the form of the infamous pre-frontal lobotomy, also became popular around this time and consisted of the removal of the prefrontal lobes of the brain, initially performed by inserting an icepick through the eye socket to dislodge the gray matter (Porter, 2002, Scull, 2015); the procedure had mixed results but often rendered the patients docile and intellectually impaired. The gruesomeness of shock treatments and ECT was depicted in books and movies and that, along with the knowledge that the procedures were administered normally without he patient's consent, was met with a societal backlash—unfortunately not before many of these were performed, however.

Early substance abuse "treatments"

As mentioned earlier in this book, most people who were addicted to alcohol and other drugs were not "treated" but punished, and they found their way into jails and poor houses. When the medical establishment of the eighteen-century adopted the idea that alcoholism was a disease that could be cured, hospitalized addicts received a series of methods which, like mental illness, consisted of bloodletting (through lancing or leeching), blistering, as well as practices to inducing vomiting, perspiration, and fear. Again, Benjamin Rush was a key practitioner of these methods, however, his refusal to adopt less aggressive methods would result in a loss of patients.

Today's treatment methods are certainly more humane and effective than those of earlier eras. There are many current models of treatment, far too many to cover in this book. We will review a few of them now.

CONTEMPORARY MENTAL HEALTH TREATMENT APPROACHES

Mental health treatment is provided in hospitals, outpatient clinics, day treatment programs, and various other venues, and is provided in individual, group, and family settings using many different treatment modalities. The term "treatment modality" refers to the specific method (or model) of treatment being employed with theoretical underpinnings that have been researched to ascertain its effectiveness. While some types of therapy are oriented toward different populations—such as children, people with borderline personality disorder, or people with religious preferences—therapeutic modalities are often available for most populations, although some are more appropriate than others for various groups. The following modalities—psychodynamic models, cognitive behavioral therapy, brief treatment models, family therapy, group therapy, and mindfulness models—are some widely used psychotherapy treatments modalities; there are many more, but these are currently favored forms and we will view these now.

Psychodynamic therapy

Sigmund Freud is arguably the name most associated with psychotherapy. He created psychoanalysis (originally hyphenated as "psycho-analysis") as a means of helping his patients uncover the unconscious motives that were causing mental distress. Psychoanalysis was the prominent model of therapy from the 1940s until the 1970s (Fancher, 1995) and it was a theoretical approach to mental illness as well as a treatment modality. His original formulation of psychoanalysis evolved into other models such as object relations therapy, interpersonal therapy, and individual psychology. To understand the current therapeutic model generally known as psychodynamic therapy, it is best to understand the early, original form known as Freudian psychoanalysis.

Many of us are familiar with certain terms and concepts associated with psychoanalysis such as the components of the personality—the id, ego, and superego; the Oedipus and Electra complexes; penis envy, and the stages of psychosexual development—the oral, anal, phallic, latency, and genital phases. Many people associate psychoanalysis with these concepts and see it as an unscientific relic of the past. However, it was, for a large portion of the twentieth century, the dominant theoretical and clinical model of mental health treatment. We will now look at the beginnings of psychoanalysis before proceeding to its current iterations of psychodynamic therapy.

An Austrian physician who had originally planned to be a researcher, Freud turned his emphasis to neurology. His scientific interests were obvious as he began to seek ways to find what was causing his patients' emotional turmoil. At the time "hysteria" was blamed for most behavioral problems, certainly for women. He began to hypothesize that perhaps the problems were a result of conflicts that existed below the level of normal consciousness, or awareness. In France, some scientists were experimenting with the use of hypnosis to cure hysteria and Freud adopted the practice as he thought it might reveal some clues about how to find the hidden find the problems that lay within the recesses of the mind. Hypnosis became a bit of a sideshow at the time, and Freud decided that having the patient talk about the issues in the form of free association, in which the patient was asked questions that required a rapid response and revealing the conflicts that exist in the unconscious parts of the mind was a preferable approach. This use of talk therapy is certainly common to us now but was not common prior to Freud, because as was discussed earlier, people with mental problems were primarily locked away in hospitals and received little therapy (Kline, 1984).

In the therapy room, Freud sat behind patients who were reclining on a couch and asked them to say the first thing that came into their minds after receiving certain prompts from the therapist. Through free association patients divulged information that he thought led to the hidden, unconscious thoughts that would reveal the real problems causing their distress. This information, however, was believed to be camouflaged in symbolism, symbolism that can be found in dreams. It can also be found in what are commonly called Freudian slips, when a faux pas occurs that exposes some hidden meaning. The therapist can analyze the disclosed information and provide the patient with insight, and through this insight, the patient will find symptom relief.

Patients, Freud determined, will often not disclose painful feelings easily. Resistance occurs which threatens the treatment, as a series of defense mechanisms are engaged to protect the vulnerable psyche. Classic psychoanalysis provides many such defenses, such as:

- *sublimation,* the most prominent method, describes when people repress unacceptable impulses and channel them to ones that are socially acceptable

Several other defenses were developed by Freud's daughter, Anna:

- *denial* happens when someone simply refuses to accept unconscious thoughts or feelings
- *repression* occurs when the patient blocks painful memories or thoughts by pushing them deeper into the unconscious
- *reaction-formation* occurs when someone reacts in the opposite way of their unconscious drives due to fear of social rejection or ridicule
- *rationalization* refers to justifying certain actions or desires that elicit feelings of guilt or social sanctions
- *projection* is the attribution of undesirable thoughts and feelings that someone possesses to other people, rather than accept those thoughts and feelings as being one's own

These defense mechanisms reflect personal defenses against instinctual drives and basically create character traits in people (Kline, 1984).

Mentioned earlier were the three components of the personality. The id is the part of the personality that is pleasure-seeking and works toward fulfilling basic needs. The superego, commonly called the conscience, is basically developed through social interaction. Unchecked, the id and superego will present problems within the individual and it is the function of the third component, the ego, to act as a regulator and prevent problems involving an excess of id or superego. A person is said to have ego strength if the ego is properly functioning.

Another key component of the clinical application of psychoanalysis are the related issues of transference and countertransference. Transference refers to the patient's identification of the therapist with some other person who figured prominently in the patient's development, often someone who positively or negatively affected the patient. Transference is an important part of therapy in that it allows the person to appropriately reflect on that person, however, it can cause strain in the therapist/client relationship if not handled appropriately. Countertransference is the other bookend to transference and refers to the therapist identifying the patient with someone in their own lives. Again, care must be taken in situations where countertransference is evident; psychoanalytically trained therapists undergo psychoanalysis themselves to realize their own unconscious thoughts and actions and how they interfere with therapy—especially regarding transference and countertransference issues.

Currently, psychodynamic therapists adhere to some of the clinical aspects above, sometimes in adapted form. They are trained to:

- develop certain skills, such as reflecting upon the patient's feelings
- determine inner psychic conflicts
- interpret, through free association and other methods, unconscious thoughts and feelings
- ascertain defense mechanisms and their meanings (Frederickson, 1999).

Due to the changes in therapy and insurance requirements, which required a change from the long, expensive psychoanalysis, newer forms have emerged in recent years such as brief psychodynamic therapy, which uses more focused, short term techniques.

Many of Freud's ideas no longer make up the main model of psychotherapy practiced today, in fact, his work seems to find more interest in the academic disciplines of theoretical psychology, sociology, and others where Freudianism is pondered and analyzed within different frameworks. Freud remains one of history's great thinkers, however, and his legacy in understanding the human mind and its relationship to society is assured (Engel, 2008).

Cognitive-behavioral therapy

Cognitive-behavioral therapy has been growing in popularity for decades. It uses components of both cognitive theory, which focuses on thought processes, and behaviorism, which focuses on action, to create a highly systematic and formulaic model of treatment. The basic idea is that maladaptive behaviors, like functional ones, are learned. According to this model, through a process of reformulating faulty thought patterns, the changing of behaviors will also occur. The changed thought patterns result in better outcomes, such as a reduction in levels of anxiety, depression, obsessive compulsive symptomology, craving for drugs, etc. Much of the treatment involves the therapist teaching the client new skills in understanding and reacting to different thoughts, feelings, and actions. In contrast with psychodynamic therapy, which primarily tries to delve into the unconscious to find the source of trouble and use the insight gained by the patient to correct the problems, the cognitive-behavioral model has numerous goals, objectives, assignments, and techniques in its treatment of people with mental health problems (Carr and McNulty 2006). We will first look at the perspective of mental illness from the perspective of the theory before moving into a discussion of treatment effects.

Most people who have taken an introductory psychology course remember the concept of operant conditioning. Operant conditioning occurs when challenging behaviors are maintained through positive reinforcement—when the behavior is rewarded and more likely to reoccur, and negative reinforcement—when situations that create distress are avoided. The primary proposition in behaviorist psychology is that people's behavior is governed to a large part by the responses—positive or negative—of others.

Cognitive theories introduce the idea that in addition to behavior, there should be a focus on cognition, which refers to all the mental processes that provide understandings of the world around us, or more basically, our consciousness. Cognitions include thoughts and other mental activity that arise out of our experiences of the world. The concept of "schema" is important in cognitive therapy and refers to a framework or mental image that organizes information for understanding objects, phenomena, or people. Incorrect information about people or things leads to "cognitive distortions", such as thoughts of personal failure, that lead to the maintenance of certain maladaptive behaviors.

A combination of these two earlier models is called cognitive behavioral therapy. The goal of treatment is to find the automatic but negative thoughts and make them known to the patient through "thought catching"—bringing attention to these thoughts and defining more adaptive patterns of thoughts and behavior, which will in turn increase emotional satisfaction. Patients will enter into a therapeutic contract with a very specific and well-defined agenda with goals specifically tailored to the patient. A host of strategies to reveal cognitive distortions are components of cognitive treatment including:

- homework assignments
- consistent feedback
- thought records
- cost-benefit analyses (Nichols and Schwartz, 2001).

Other strategies that make up the behavioral component of cognitive-behavioral therapy include:

- negative thought stopping exercises
- distraction techniques
- physical activity
- communication skill building techniques
- relaxation exercises (Nichols and Schwartz, 2001).

There are many modified forms of CBT, or methodologies that are closely aligned with many of its basic tenets. One of the most noteworthy is rational-emotive behavior therapy (REBT), developed by Albert Ellis (1978) and that uses the well-known ABC method of explaining to client how activating events (A), often create an irrational belief (B) about the action, that eventually leads to a consequence (C); since how a certain action is interpreted is what is important, clients are taught to try to develop skills in interpretation and how to deal with bothersome cognitions. Dialectical behavior therapy (DBT), created in the 1980s, is a form of treatment often used with people with personality disorders, those with addictions, eating disorders and depression, that encourages self-regulation of their responses to emotional triggers (Chapman, 2006). Acceptance and commitment therapy (ACT) is also a modality from the 1980s which attempts to help clients to better understand the cognitive problems they are experiencing, but rather than to force cognitive change, they are taught to accept the situation, often using mindfulness therapy techniques to accomplish this end (Dualdiagnosis.org, 2018).

Brief models of therapy

The term brief psychotherapy encompasses several different types of treatment models that seek to keep therapy short, focused, and in the present. The impracticality and inefficacy of long-term, expensive treatment that was a factor in psychoanalytic treatment and other extensive programs, began being questioned beginning as early as the 1940s but came into full bloom decades later when Health Management Organizations (HMO's) started regulating the number and type of therapy sessions that were available for people under insurance plans. Guided by the HMO changes, brief therapy aligned with these changes with these expectations:

- therapy is to be directed toward specific problems with goals to seek symptom resolution
- therapy reflects a rapid response and has a crisis preparedness orientation;
- therapy has a specific and time limited contract
- treatment planning will allow flexible meetings
- treatment adopts an eclectic perspective that includes other treatment modalities, including psychopharmacology
- an intermittent treatment format is maintained that allows the client to return for treatment later for other problems (the "family practitioner model")

- and an accountability and oversight component is developed to ensure the treatment provided was effective and efficient (Hoyt, 2003).

Clinicians who employ brief therapy often see the information gained from an assessment as a narrative of the person's life. This biography is used to ascertain the role of family life circumstances and family resources that can be utilized and to create and prioritize goals (Lane, 2000). Many brief-oriented therapists also seek out client strengths as well as challenges and incorporate these assets into the treatment process. There are many benefits to reducing the amount of time spent in treatment:

- the prioritization of therapy goals which naturally occurs in this modality
- the more effective use of energy directed toward the goals deems most important
- the amount of money spent
- the fact that some clients have a limited period of treatment due to upcoming relocation (physical move, ending of school terms, job transfer, etc.)
- the fact that when time is a valued resource people are often more productive, as opposed to an on-going process where no immediate end is in sight (Phillips, 1985).
- the value of time limitations is important in creating boundaries which provide a form of safety, security, and parameters of treatment (Mander, 2000).

In addition, brief counseling is focused on problem resolution in that it relies on client strengths and aspirations to guide treatment. It is also action-based, as it focuses on removing barriers that keep people in problematic thoughts and behaviors. It is socially interactive as it seeks patient engagement in meaningful social relationships. Brief treatment focuses on concrete, rather than vague and abstract thoughts and feelings, and attends to developmental ages and transitions. Humor is often invoked to move beyond client pain and to develop positive emotions. The stance of the brief therapist is warm and empathetic, as opposed to distant or authoritative (Littrell, 1998). Therefore, brief therapy, in its different forms, is future-focused and emphasizes concrete ways to resolve problematic thoughts, feelings, and behaviors.

There are several models of brief therapy. One of the most noted is solution-focused brief therapy (SFBT), or simply solution-focused therapy.

This type of therapy, as the name implies, is concerned with the outcomes of treatment and emphasizes solutions to the problems patients are encountering. It is closely identified with family therapy and a specific family therapy modality known as strategic therapy. Solution-focused brief therapy sees the therapeutic relationship as being one of collaboration between therapist and client, and due to this collaboration, the outcomes are viewed as being co-created.

There are some key figures in this treatment model, but none looms as large as Milton Erickson who developed his model in the period from the late 1920s to the late 1970s. Departing from the prevalent model of psychoanalysis, Erickson was less concerned with the reason for the presenting problem than how to bring about change; thus, he cared little about theory, focusing his attention on many techniques to promote change through solutions (O'Hanlon & Weiner-Davis, 1989).

Therefore, in SFBT, there is an emphasis on the strengths of patients to help solve their own problems, in conjunction with the therapist. SFBT has many strategies and intriguing concepts to bring about change in patients such as:

- providing "solution talk", in which clients are encouraged to use talk that engages solutions rather than "problem talk"
- "reframing", to propose a new, and more positive, interpretation of what is considered a problem event
- finding "exceptions", in which patients recall and analyze times when the problem events did not exist to provide insight into possible solutions
- "externalizing" problem situations by relocating them from the person (in which the problems were earlier internalized) to a problem on its own to be solved
- "scaling", or placing troubling feelings, thoughts, or behaviors on a scale, or continuum, for better examination and solution seeking
- pondering the "miracle question" which asks clients to imagine a situation in which the problems don't exist and to describe this image so together the therapist and client can find solutions to get to that result (Winbolt, 2011)

Another model of the brief-oriented genre is narrative therapy, which evolved in the 1990s, and focuses on the communication process in which patients construct meaning and make sense of their problems. Patients, like everyone else, have "problem saturated stories" and in narrative therapy these stories are examined and redefined into different, more productive perspectives. The use of metaphors is often used to analyze and bring about the more beneficial narratives. Communication in its metaphorical state can unleash the imagination and inspire patients to make positive changes in several ways:

- metaphor has the dual capability to create rapid insight but also promote a sustained processing of information
- metaphor in narratives has veiled insights which are sometimes received as less threatening than the use of direct comments, which can be confrontational and can result in patient resistance
- metaphors allow the unconscious thoughts to surface for closer analysis and greater insights (in this way it resembles psychodynamic models)
- patients can use metaphors to construct their own understanding of what the story means and how it relates to their own presenting problems
- the revealing of unconscious thoughts reduces the level of resistance that comes from excessively rational thought (after all, it is just a story)
- the flexibility of story-telling in the form of metaphor promotes different opinions and the ability to reframe if needed—the possibility of creating a "different story" with better outcomes
- metaphors also allow for projection of thoughts and behaviors (again, sounding a little like psychodynamic therapy) to a person in a story which makes undesirable thoughts or feelings more available for analysis—this is like the solution-focused concept of externalization except the external object in narrative therapy exists in the story
- the value of metaphors, while beneficial to adults, can be especially beneficial to children who are used to hearing and reading fables and tales; this sharing can reinforce rapport with adult practitioners
- metaphors can contribute to the cultural aspects of storytelling which can be used by therapists who provide clinical supervision and mentorship to students and novice practitioners (Barker, 1985)

Family therapy

Family therapy, often called marriage and family therapy, is a therapeutic model that seeks to include treatment of whole families (at least as many that will attend therapy sessions). Family therapy, is relatively new, beginning around the 1950s as a defined, established practice, though finding a specific date or originator is difficult. The idea of working with entire families to address the mental health needs of at least one of its members extends much earlier than this, however. For example, social work, which was formed in the late 1800s as an outgrowth of charity programs in the United States and England, occurred often within the context of family work. In addition, the child guidance movement which began just after the turn of the twentieth century and grew, albeit slowly, to cities across the United States, also was a major force in planting the seeds of doing therapy with families. Another movement that was responsible for the turn to family therapy was the group counseling movement, which looked to fostering interpersonal communications between people to improve healthy relationships (Nichols & Swartz, 2001).

More direct roots can be found in a large research program on families with schizophrenic members; the "schizophrenogenic mother" was a major focus with this endeavor, echoing the blame placed on women for family problems (and psychological problems generally at mid-twentieth century) This research program, beginning in the 1940s, sought to understand communication patterns in families, obviously more problematic in schizophrenic families, and brought together a host of scholars from different fields, such as cultural anthropology, social psychology, communication, and psychiatry. These scholars and practitioners broke with the tradition of treating family members separately, which in the era of psychoanalysis was a requirement. As time progressed, an interest in working with entire families began and a new form of therapy was born.

Family therapy incorporates the same modalities as mentioned earlier—psychodynamic, cognitive-behavioral, brief, and the others mentioned in this section, however, family therapy has its own sub-modalities specific to family treatment such as family systems therapy, structural family therapy, and strategic approaches. There are different subtypes of family systems therapy, but all involve treating the family system; while individual treatment models have an "identified patient", in systemic models, the family is the identified patient. Perhaps the most prominent model of family systems therapy is the Bowenian model, named after its founder Murray Bowen. This formulation plays close attention to how problems in families are passed down to the succeeding generations and the extent to which family members are differentiated, meaning how they achieve healthy separation from other members. Bowenian therapy also posits that stress in families creates the need to bring in another person, a process called triangulation, to reduce the level of stress. Bowenian systems therapy seeks to promote active differentiation in families, detriangulation, and stress reduction. Due to the focus on the transmission of family problems to following families, systems therapists (as well as other family practitioners) uses a genogram—basically a clinical family tree—which exposes problems originating in previous generations that are causing current emotional distress (Nichols & Swartz, 2001).

Another form of family therapy is known as structural family therapy and was developed primarily by Salvador Minuchin, who like Bowen was a psychiatrist originally trained in psychoanalytic therapy. Minuchin, however, worked with institutionalized youth and inner-city families and perceived of family problems as developing from inappropriate structures, or the ways in which families are organized; these structures set up interaction patterns that can be destructive to the family unit. If family structure is at fault—for example, if the boundaries are too rigid or too flexible, or if members form subsystems that are unhealthy or conflictual—the result is a dysfunctional family organization. In structural family therapy, the therapist joins with the family in an active way and seeks to promote a more structured family environment (Nichols & Swartz, 2001).

Strategic family therapy can be traced to three major sources, two in America and the other in Italy. In America, it can be traced back to late 1950s to the early researchers of the Mental Research Institute (MRI) who sought to understand the role of communication in families, especially those with a schizophrenic family member. Other American therapists further developed "paradoxical interventions", in which reverse psychology strategies are used to modify the behavior of family members. A group of therapists in Milan, Italy who were impressed by the early theoretical progress of the America model, continued the development of this type of therapy by using male/female co-therapists, having another group of therapists observing the therapy sessions, and creating novel techniques. All three of the models in the strategic vein, are extremely formulaic and governed by techniques. And all three seek pragmatic ways to elicit change in problematic sequences of family behavior. As mentioned earlier, strategic therapy was one of the forerunners of brief, solution-focused models; strategic therapy uses active engagement of the therapists to promote change.

Families have certainly changed since the formal establishment of family therapy in the 1950s, a time considered by some to be the "golden era" of family life, an idea which has been exposed as a myth (Coontz, 1992). Families are different today as newer societal ideas have developed about what constitutes family. In addition, economic and technological forces have created many changes since the therapy's early days. Therapists practicing family treatment must be mindful of the continually changing family institution and with the changes in family therapeutic models.

Group therapy

Group therapy, as the name implies, refers to counseling sessions that take place within a setting with other people experiencing (often similar) problems and that seeks to bring about positive change in the group members. It usually has a group leader who facilitates the group in discussion on certain topics or general ones, but that pertains to shared experiences of the group. Group treatment can be led by a professional therapist or by a non-clinically trained person who has an active and engaged role in the focus of the group; AA, for example normally uses a member without clinical training as the leader. Therapy groups come in different sizes—from large to small, although smaller groups usually tend to be more effective. The group can take place in institutional or outpatient settings. Group therapy programs utilize a large variety of treatment modalities such as those listed in this section, while others, such as psychoeducation groups (whose purpose is to educate rather than treat) are used in prevention programs.

Early efforts at working with individuals in a group format have been seen by some scholars as beginning as far back as ancient Greece (in the form of the Greek Drama), to the medieval period (in the morality play), or in the eighteenth century (in the form of mesmerism). A more likely beginning for modern professional group work can be found in the early 20th century in the practice of physicians working with patients with tuberculosis, schizophrenia, and manic-depressive disorders. A defined version of group psychology developed after World War I and produced such group therapy terms and concepts as "herd instinct" and "group mind" (Klein, Bernard, & Singer, 1992). Initially using a lecture-type format, group therapy was lauded for its practicality due to its potential for disclosing information to groups (even large ones) simultaneously, saving time, energy, and money, as staffing costs were less and people who were unable to pay for institutional or individual treatment were able to afford group meetings (Dies, 2003); which in some contexts, such as AA, were, and continue to be, free.

One of the key figures in group therapy was Kurt Lewin whose work in social psychology was the impetus for the T-group method (the "T" stands for training) which started prior to World War II. T-groups were created in organizational settings to assist workers to better understand each other. Other treatment providers followed this format including therapists who were being trained to provide counseling to soldiers returning from war—

these group methods came to be later used by their creator, Carl Rogers, to develop encounter groups. Encounter groups were based on his humanistic, client-oriented approach to therapy, and focused on several key elements:

- openness
- acceptance
- honesty
- feedback
- disclosure
- participant observation
- empathetic understanding (Rogers, 1970; Klein, Bernard, & Singer, 1992).

This soul-searching type of group therapy flourished in the 1960s and 1970s when social and political causes were popular (Spitz & Spitz, 1999). Another antecedent to group treatment was a form of spontaneous play which its founder, Jacob Moreno, named psychodrama and produced the familiar role-playing technique which is a component of certain forms of group psychotherapy (Shaffer & Galinsky, 1989).

Group therapy's early roots in psychoeducation were replaced when its therapeutic value became obvious to the group leaders. The experiences of the members, when shared with the group, who in turn shared their stories with others, often produced a degree of catharsis, or psychological comfort. Mental health professionals, pleased with the results, continued to expand group counseling, and eventually, this modality began to adopt different theoretical and therapeutic underpinnings. Early on, psychoanalysis in its ascendency filled this role, even though some of its more individualistic components are incompatible with group work (Dies, 2003). Later, most of the other major treatment modalities would incorporate group treatment into their practice.

Group treatment in outpatient settings is normally scheduled weekly, often in one and one-half hour segments, though the time increments may vary. Group work in institutional environments is provided more regularly than in outpatient settings—often several times per week or even daily. They are also more likely to have ancillary activities such as recreation and occupational programs, dramatic performances, and alternative group arrangements. As brief forms of therapy continue to direct mental health treatment, group work tends to concentrate on certain goals:

- relief of symptoms
- self-esteem building
- relationship skill building
- problem-solving skill enhancement
- peer acceptance competencies (Dies, 2003).

Groups may be open-ended, in which new members are added when others depart or closed, in which a peer cohort is maintained, with no new members entering the group. Open-ended groups tend to be less stable than closed groups due to their constant fluctuations (which require re-establishing trust and group norms) but they have the advantages of enhancing adjustment and coping skills. Closed groups, while having limited use in longer term therapy, can focus on treatment rather than the assimilation processes required of continually changing groups (Dies, 2003).

Group therapy envisions a series of stages through which the group progresses. There have been many such formulations of this type of mental health treatment and different stage progressions, but the following provides a good representation of the general stage process of group work:

1. The initial stage of "forming, storming, norming, and performing" (using this wonderful alliteration by Tuckman, 1965), issues of social anxiety and trust exist as patients try to interpret the other members' thoughts and actions.
2. The conflict stage is marked by discord and frustration as members try to assert independence while seeking safety and validation.
3. The cohesion stage in which bonding occurs between the group members due to increased familiarity and trust and where less leadership is provided by the facilitator.
4. The final stage of termination when members are expected to use skills learned in the group in their lives outside the group; this stage often includes emotions of sadness and apprehension about leaving the group (Brown, 2013).

Group psychotherapy has many benefits in that it:

- allows clients to see themselves as other group members see them
- provides insight into the motivations and personality characteristics of others

- promotes an understanding of power dynamics and the inducements of conformity
- gives experience in dealing with interpersonal stress (Halleck, 1971)

Mindfulness approaches

Mindfulness is a new approach in the mental health treatment field, at least as a formalized mode of Western psychotherapy (philosophically its Eastern roots are much deeper). Mindfulness is a core feature of Buddhist philosophy and refers to a state of awareness in which the here-and-now prevails over the experiences of the past, as well as the potential conflicts that may arise in the future. The word is a translation of the early Indian language *pali* and refers not only to awareness, but also sustained attention and remembering (Germer, 2013).

The perceived potential of Eastern philosophy as a supplement to Western psychotherapy, while currently very much in vogue, is not new. William James, the seminal philosopher-psychologist scholar of the late nineteenth and early twentieth centuries, believed this integration would occur by the mid-twentieth century. Carl Jung, psychoanalyst and disciple of Freud (who would later break away from the master), maintained a fascination with Eastern religion, as can be found in many of his writings. Other psychoanalysts such as Erich Fromm and Karen Horney adopted these foreign ideas into their interpretations of psychotherapy. After World War II, the philosophies of the East, especially Zen Buddhism, became a part of Western culture as it attracted the interests of many intellectuals, writers, and visionaries (Epstein, 1995, Germer, 2013).

In recent years, mindfulness has become incorporated into the mainstream mental health landscape. It is popular due to many factors, such as its transtheoretical nature, meaning it is used across theoretical orientations and treatment modalities. It is also transdiagnostic, in that it seems to have positive effects on a wide variety of disorders and conditions (Germer, 2013). In mindfulness therapy, meditation is used to produce the awareness needed to reduce anxiety by re-focusing attention from a materialistic, narcissism-creating world to one that focuses on the appreciation and validation of internal feelings of acceptance and compassion of self and others. Therapists are encouraged to personally use mindfulness practices and to model them for clients (MacDonald, 2016).

It is easy to see the concerns that exist over the scientific validity of a modality that is based on a philosophical notion. It is difficult to subject meditative states and their intrapsychic effects to scientific scrutiny (MacDonald, 2016). Results from a recent review of research (Davis &

Hayes, 2011), however, suggests mindfulness therapy has positive effects in emotion regulation, resulting from improved cognitive enhancement; interpersonal relationships; and physical and emotional well-being. In addition, therapists who use and model mindfulness can receive enhanced skills involved in empathy, compassion, and general counseling techniques (Davis & Hayes, 2011). This model of therapy is presently very popular in the psychotherapy field not only as a freestanding modality but also as a major component of other treatments such as dialectical behavioral therapy and acceptance and commitment therapy.

CONTEMPORARY SUBSTANCE ABUSE TREATMENT

Substance abuse treatment occurs in a variety of settings—institutional, outpatient, and group. Therapists trained in addictions treatment need to understand not only aspects of mental health but also drugs of abuse and their effects, the addiction process, addictive behavior, cravings, relapse, recovery, and triggers that are related to drugs and other addictions. Since many acts involving alcohol and other drugs involve criminal behavior, substance abuse treatment is often connected with the criminal justice system, therefore, the issue of court-ordered or other mandated treatment is a common issue in treatment considerations.

Many of the mental health models mentioned before are used in substance abuse treatment so there is no one model that practitioners use—some may use a primarily psychodynamic approach, a mindfulness approach, family therapy, brief models, or a combination of these or other modalities. However, currently the cognitive-behavioral approach appears to show the most promise because of its benefits in changing illogical thinking, which is often a key issue in the addiction process. Group treatment is also a major component of addictions counseling because of the advantages in hearing the experiences of other addicted people that can serve as a guide for their own behavior. Family therapy can be advantageous in families with addiction to uncover and address issues such as codependency, in which family members adjust in maladaptive ways in dealing with the addiction of one or more members of the family.

Many models of substance abuse treatment utilize a strict abstinence approach such as the "self-help" types based on the Alcoholics Anonymous (AA) model. AA programs are often called twelve step programs as they offer a series of twelve steps that are to be followed to promote the maintenance of sobriety. Many are familiar with the story of two men, William G. Wilson and Robert H. Smith, the founders of AA. Wilson (better known as Bill W.) was a businessman who had suffered from depression and later alcohol addiction. Smith (Dr. Bob), was a physician who also suffered from alcoholism since college and who, incidentally received his medical education at Rush Medical College (named after Benjamin Rush). In 1935, Bill W. was away from home and in need of someone to talk to and he feared a relapse. He contacted Dr. Bob, whom he did not know, and the two worked together to create a program to help other addicted people. They published the "Big Book", outlining their ideas of total abstinence and group support to resist drug use (Fletcher, 2013). Other substance abuse programs that have followed the lead of AA are Narcotics Anonymous (NA), Cocaine Anonymous (CA), and some that deal with behavioral conditions such as Gamblers Anonymous (GA), Overeaters Anonymous, and Sexaholics Anonymous (SA). These models normally follow the premise that substance addiction is a disease and that any use of the substance during the recovery stage will create a relapse, setting the cycle in motion again. The idea of powerlessness, a central theme and addressed in the first of the twelve steps, has distinct meanings in American culture as the use of addictive substances (as an exaggerated form of consumption) exposes long term understandings of power relations (Cushman, 1995). Therefore, the self-help models, as many other substance use treatments, rely heavily on the concepts of relapse prevention and recovery. These programs often use the group format.

An alternative to the twelve step programs is the harm reduction model, mentioned earlier, which accepts the fact that most people who are addicted to drugs relapse, the goal, therefore, is to minimize the damage when relapse occurs. This approach assumes that total abstinence is not a reality for most drug abusers and is supported by the "stages of change model" (Prochaska & DiClemente, 1982) which posits five stages:

1. The precontemplation stage, in which the addicted person has no intention of changing the using behavior
2. The contemplation stage, in which the person actively considers discontinuing drug use
3. The preparation stage, in which motivation to change is backed up with preparation
4. The action stage, in which the person makes the change
5. The maintenance stage where relapse prevention is sustained

Harm reduction interventions assume that many people who would avoid abstinence models will be able to make some positive attempts at recovery (MacMaster, 2004). Since drug policy and most addiction perspectives stress zero tolerance, harm reduction runs counter to this orientation and is controversial for this reason (MacMaster, 2004).

In addition to the concepts of abstinence and relapse, the issue of the motivation to use addictive substances has become a major focus of treatment in the last few decades. The intentions of addicted people to remain abstinent and not succumb to relapse is attributable to the motivations, both internal and external, that guide their behavior. A technique called motivational interviewing, a relatively new method that was developed to thwart problem drinking, merged with the brief therapy approach and uses the stages of change model as a guide to promote abstinence. Motivational interviewing is a strategy that ensures that clients are provided with a safe environment to confront their own ambivalence (internal motivations) toward making the changes needed for an addiction-free lifestyle (Miller & Rollick, 2002). Another strategy known as contingency management seeks to address motivation from an external standpoint. Based on operant conditioning concepts, rewards such as vouchers that can be used as valued gifts are provided to clients who refrain from drug use. In a recent review of the research, Sayegh, Huey, Zara, and Jhaveri (2017) suggest both motivational interviewing and contingency management approaches are generally effective in increasing motivational efforts to abstain from drug use.

A cornucopia of different treatment approaches

As can be seen, mental health practitioners have a wide variety of different treatment strategies with which to assist clients. While some therapists work within a particular framework, there are many different models that are available. Obviously, some therapists work better within some frameworks than others, but sometimes an integrated approach is used which pulls from different modalities to create a treatment program that is deemed to be the most beneficial to the client. Treatment populations such as children, racial and ethnic minorities, LGBTQ patients, the disabled, and others might need a different approach than is often used; therapists must make these issues into consideration when adopting a model for therapy.

Therapeutic models rise and fall in popularity. Currently, mindfulness therapy and acceptance and commitment therapy are very popular in the therapy field. As times change, new therapies grow in popularity, others will fall out of favor, while others will stand the test of time. And many will become modified or merge with others.

Despite the vast array of treatment modalities at the therapist's disposal, eminent therapist Irvin D. Yalom (1989) sees the relationship between the therapist and client as having the most beneficial outcomes on therapy; as Yalom states that "this encounter, the very heart of psychotherapy, is a caring, deeply human meeting between two people, one (generally, but not always, the patient) more troubled than the other" (Yalom, 1989, p.13). He notes the dual role of the therapist—as both observer and participant—and explains the therapeutic relationship as a deeply moving and transformational relationship to both parties.

CONCLUSION

The methods used to "treat" mental illness has a storied past. The mad were bled, blistered, had their bowels evacuated, forced to vomit and sweat, dunked, frightened, incarcerated, restrained in shackles, shocked, lobotomized, beaten, hypnotized, magnetized, sterilized, drugged, and had their heads drilled. They were also subjected to a strange assortment of what would today seem to be torture devices. These methods were used in attempts to relieve suffering and to protect the public from their behavior.

Much has changed since that time and many forms of psychotherapy have emerged. Psychodynamic models have been in use for several decades. Psychoanalysis enjoyed prominence in the early to the mid-twentieth century, not only as a therapeutic technique but also a theoretical framework which became pervasive in the general culture; however, due to changes in healthcare and the mental health field (not to mention society generally), psychoanalysis lost prominence, and became replaced with other models. Cognitive-behavioral therapy provides a very scientific, short-term, clinical option and is still a mainstay in therapy. Other brief, solution-oriented models, family therapy, group therapy, and practices that involve the Eastern philosophy of mindfulness, have also offered significant benefits to those needing therapy. Therapists do indeed have many therapeutic options, but in the end, the words of Irvin Yalom might provide some insight—the heart of psychotherapy lies in the relationship between therapist and client.

The therapeutic substructure that supports the current modalities in psychotherapy suggests that we believe that therapy contains an element of both intuition and empirical rationalization; in other words, therapy is seen as both art and science. This can be realized in the fact that we have many different models of therapy—if there wasn't a belief in different styles for different therapists, there would be a "one-size-fits-all" approach that all therapists would practice. Even in view of research data on certain modalities, it is still up to the therapist to decide the treatment model to be used. The cultural value attached to the therapist's personal characteristics to promote positive change should alleviate fears that technology will soon take over the task of psychotherapy's healers.

Chapter 5

THE SOCIOLOGICAL PERSPECTIVE

> "...we deem that the sociologist will not have completed his mission so long as he has not penetrated the inmost depths of individuals, in order to relate to their psychological condition the instructions of which he gives an account"
>
> (Emile Durkheim 1909/1982, p. 236).

USING THE SOCIOLOGICAL IMAGINATION TO UNDERSTAND MENTAL ILLNESS

In the last chapter, we examined the mental health system from a psychotherapeutic perspective. In this chapter, we will look at the system from a sociological perspective, noting the contributions of this discipline, particularly theoretical formulations to the field. We will examine the thoughts and works of scholars who took a sociological perspective in understanding mental health and mental illness. Although some of these ideas were produced by sociologists—Erich Fromm, Erving Goffman, and Thomas Scheff (and to a lesser degree we will examine the ideas of sociologists C. Wright Mills, Emile Durkheim, Karl Marx, George Herbert Mead, and Max Weber), other sociological insights were made by psychiatrists Thomas Szasz and R.D. Laing, social philosopher Michel Foucault, and psychologist D.L. Rosenhan. The common thread of the ideas of these thinkers is the critical approach used to better understand mental illness, which required a way of "thinking outside the box". These ideas will be considered with contrasting ideas.

Sociologist C. Wright Mills was a maverick who offered scathing critiques of American society. He was a public intellectual who became well-known in and outside academic circles and was especially noted for his work on the problems of modern life, focusing primarily on political concerns. However, late in his career he published a more reflective work that bore the name of a what would become a standard tool used to analyze society—*The Sociological Imagination* (1959). He described how people are trapped in modern society, a society in need of close analysis to effectively treat social problems. It takes the use of imagination to see how the mental health "troubles" of individuals are connected to the social "issues" of war, unemployment, inequality, and rapid urbanization. Conflicts can be viewed from both the personal and social levels, or, as he put it, biography (a person's story) and history (a society's story): "the life of an individual cannot be adequately understood without references to the institutions within which his biography is enacted" (Mills, 1959, p.161).

Written in the late 1950s, *The Sociological Imagination* describes a world in which is changing so rapidly a person's individual biography has different adaptations to the "historical push and shove" (Mills, 1959, p. 6), referring to the social conditions that move people in ways they cannot handle or often predict. The result is a social malaise, or anxiety (note that these terms, malaise and anxiety, are also used to describe individual pathologies as well as social ones). Turning to the field to psychoanalysis, Mills asserted the analysts were wrong in positing that problems arise from the "dark forces" in the human psyche; instead he stated that the genesis of personal problems could be found in the "unruly forces of contemporary society itself, with its alienating methods of production, its enveloping techniques of political domination, its international anarchy—in a word, its pervasive transformation of the very 'nature' of man and the conditions and aims of his life" (Mills, 1959, p.13). History must be examined and revised to make lasting changes in our individual biographies. Mills was bothered by how social scientists, especially psychologists and psychiatrists, failed to account for the role of social factors in the treatment of individual problems—one exception he noted was Erich Fromm.

IS SOCIETY SANE? REFLECTIONS FROM ERICH FROMM

This is a question that was asked by Erich Fromm, a psychoanalyst and social theorist whose later works became popular bestsellers such as *Escape from Freedom* (1941), a psychoanalytic examination of totalitarianism, and its follow-up, *The Sane Society* (1955). Fromm obtained a Ph.D. in sociology and shortly thereafter entered training as a psychoanalyst, gaining an understanding of not only sociology but also psychology and psychiatry. Fromm joined the Frankfurt School of Critical Theory, a think tank that started in Germany but escaped Nazism to set up shop in New York at Columbia University. The group sought to understand social problems, such as Fascism, by combining the unlikely theoretical perspectives of Freudian psychoanalysis and Marxist ideology. Fromm would eventually experience a harsh break-up with the group but went on to a prolific solo writing career.

In his highly important work *The Sane Society* (1955), Fromm dispelled the idea that the world in the 20th century seemed to be the epitome of a sane society. Looking beneath the surface, he posits, one can see the contradiction—just as people who are mentally ill see themselves as sane, many "sane" people today (or in the last century when Fromm was writing) are delusional. Although the United States is the wealthiest country in the world, there is still poverty, war, and a reliance on false needs and interests which lack any true substance—he referred especially to anti-intellectual movies, television shows, and radio programs. In a footnoted passage, Fromm explained a time when he asked his college students their responses to spending three days alone with no radio or modern "escapist" literature; ninety percent said they would experience high levels of anxiety under these conditions—think of how people today would react if there were no cell phones, internet, or social media! Despite the free time we have the luxury of enjoying, Fromm stated we simply get bored. In contrast, to the claims of psychology and psychiatry that some individuals are maladjusted in a generally sane world, he stated the whole culture suffers from a "pathology of normalcy" in which those in the soft, comfortable middle classes have levels of boredom that are addressed by self-medication of alcohol, other drugs, and suicide (Fromm, 1955).

Echoing C. Wright Mills, Fromm states "just as man transforms the world around him, so he transforms himself in the process of history" (Fromm, 1955, p.13). If individuals develop themselves appropriately in a culture that is accommodating to self-development, they can achieve sanity, but if the society itself is defective, sanity cannot be attained. A "socially patterned defect" occurs if many people have mental disturbances; if these "defects", such as greed, excessive ambition, vanity, power hunger, and destructiveness, become common to a culture, they are no longer a mental illness—they *are* the culture. As he notes "the culture provides patterns which enable them to live without becoming ill" (Fromm, 1955, p.16).

Fromm breaks from the Freudian convention of mental illness resulting from issues involving sexuality to issues of what he called the "human situation" (p. 28), the existential problems that result from being a human creature, whose evolutionary features have separated people from animals and from nature itself. This humanistic psychoanalytical position means that people become mentally ill when they are unable to find answers to their own existence and are unable to make connections to people, groups, organizations, institutions, or religion others that make life worth living. The way people can successfully relate to their world is through love and the key issue is the quality of the love rather than the object of affection. Without this loving connection to others, a pathology develops in the form of narcissism, which Fromm saw as being ever present in the most severe forms of mental illness (Fromm, 1955).

Fromm was understandably concerned with the problems wrought by excessive nationalism—the “fixation to blood and soil” –and he likened this to a form of incest with its cult being patriotism. As the United States and parts of Europe have experienced increasing levels of nationalism and other anti-globalist tendencies, Fromm’s ideas seem to have increased salience today.

Moving into discussions that reflects a Marxist philosophy, Fromm explained that a materialist perspective creates our conscious experiences. Using the idea of a “social character”, a concept often found in the sociological literature, Fromm states each society has a cultural function to marshal the energies of its people toward a specific goal. In highly capitalistic societies the energy needed to produce large assets of capital, goods, and services is directed in the form of punctuality and orderliness (Fromm, 1955). Therefore, again we see a connection between history and biography—social character influences individual character, that is, personality. It is the social institution of the family that conveys to the new members of society the dictates of the social character.

The social character has produced a collectivity of people who desire the goods and services created by capitalism and who are willing to function as a team working in machine fashion to keep the cogs turning; they accept the illusion they are free. Buying materials is primarily for acquisition purposes only—we buy things we don’t need, thinking these things make us free acting individuals. We are alienated, as Marx would say, to the things produced and to the whole production process itself. And, we are “consumption hungry” (Fromm, 1941, p.135) and constantly demand new gadgets—the pleasure that comes from owning the thing is greater than the thing’s true value. Interestingly, Fromm in referencing the mid-1900s discussed the seemingly recent disorder (to use his word) of hoarding—the inability to let go of material things; we can remember from chapter three that hoarding is now an official DSM-5 diagnosis. The twentieth century response to material goods is what Fromm called a “receptive orientation” (1955, p.136) in which the consumerist goal is to constantly have new things, rather than just hoarding old ones. Things themselves matter little since the fun is in the acquisition; things themselves become alien (creating “alienation”). Since things lack a self, the owner also lacks a self. This is, in Fromm’s view (and the views of other scholars such as Henry Stack Sullivan), a mental disorder. Therefore alienation, routinization, maladjustment, and a breakdown of social order (which founding sociologist Emile Durkheim called “anomie”) result in pathological states.

We now have a detailed example of a mentally disordered (insane) society, as diagnosed by Erich Fromm. His prescription included:

- a series of advances in the political, economic, and cultural spheres
- the abolishment of all forms of military action
- the institution of a world government
- global trade
- political involvement on local levels
- extended opportunities for educational attainment
- income equality
- a focus on caring for our fellow world citizens (Fromm, 1955)

As mentioned in the last chapter in the section on brief, solution-focused therapies, the strategy for happiness is to create a possibility narrative rather than a problem-saturated one. By asking the miracle question on a macro level, we can envision a bright future and specify the correct ways to approach these goals. If individual troubles must be addressed as social issues, as Mills suggested, Fromm's prescriptions are more than just utopian solutions, they will end up creating a sane society.

IS SOCIETY MAD? REFLECTIONS FROM MICHEL FOUCAULT

Michel Foucault was a French social philosopher, historian, and public intellectual whose ideas so greatly affected sociology, his work is often analyzed in postmodern and post-structural theories of society that grew in prominence during the mid- and later-twentieth century. His broad interests included incarceration, sexuality, medicine, and of course, madness. In analyzing these and other areas, he used a historical approach that paid heed to the changes and phases of the objects of study, applying a critical eye to these transitions to ascertain the great social implications represented in these changes.

One of Foucault's greatest works, *Madness and Civilization* (1988), originally published in French in 1961, explores the meanings behind the treatment of the mentally ill, primarily in Europe in three epochs:

1. The Renaissance,
2. The "classical era" of the late seventeenth and eighteenth centuries
3. The "age of the asylum".

These stages offer information regarding views and strategies—often harmful ones—that existed in Europe during these periods.

The Renaissance was a time when wisdom and knowledge were valued. The mentally ill were perceived as somehow gifted with a type of spiritual insight that revealed the chaotic nature of humankind and exposes the limits of humanity. Those with mental illness were attributed a degree of mysticism and this idea Foucault describes as being depicted in the art and literature of the period. The approaches to mental illness were certainly different from the preceding period, the Middle Ages, when the "mad" were a group that were banished to other places throughout Europe. At times, this banishment occurred in the form of sailing vessels in the so-called "ship of fools" which cast a light on the mad in the same regard as lepers. In vivid language, Foucault explained how the mentally ill are the "passenger par excellence" and notes that "water and madness have long been linked in the dreams of European men" (1988, p.12). But the Renaissance was a different time and these numinous mad persons could walk freely and were viewed with veneration. This type of treatment did not continue into the next period.

In the classical period, the mentally ill came to be viewed as a distinct social type, along with the poor, the non-working, and the criminal; in other words, an outcast. Throughout Europe, grand new constructions were erected for these former wanderers. Though called hospitals, they were not medical structures but places to house the unfortunate souls who occupied the lower strata of society, people who needed to be both hidden and controlled. Thus, the ideas that resulted from building these institutions created a new understanding of madness. This period Foucault called the Great Confinement.

The last period was the modern era when the asylum was created, and reforms were made to what had become very inhumane conditions for the mentally ill. A medical model was instituted and due to an emerging view of mental illness as sickness, a new vision of treating madness began to appear. The mad were now locked away from society to be "cured" of their disease. We can recall from chapter two, reformers such William Pinel were generally regarded as heroes in the struggle to humanize the mentally ill; Foucault was not kind to these reformers as he believed their motivations as being based more on oppression than morality.

It is important to see Foucault's argument—madness is viewed as a product of social conditions at different points of history. The mad have been perceived during the periods in Europe he described as being fools, prophets, outcasts, and eventually, as sick people in the need of medical care. *Madness and Civilization* is not as accessible as the other works mentioned in this chapter, and it has been roundly criticized for its historical inaccuracies. However, it is an important work in that it challenges the prevailing view that mental illness has always been viewed as a medical condition. It also raises questions about the exact nature of mental illness. If views of it have changed as social situations have, how stable is the concept? These questions will have been taken up by other mental health scholars and will be discussed soon.

Foucault's work ends with an analysis of the period of asylums in his historical examination of mental illness. In the 1950s and 1960s when scholars began questioning the utility of the mental hospital system, a major work on the subject appeared, a work based on actual field research at a well-known American asylum. It cast some light on the workings of these cryptic places and the curious treatment programs that were going on behind the walls. And it adopted the sociological focus on power imbalances as they have persisted in the topic of madness in a so-called civilized society.

A LOOK BEHIND THE WALLS: ERVING GOFFMAN

Erving Goffman was a Canadian-American sociologist who created seminal works in a theoretical formulation called symbolic interactionism, a micro level approach that emphasizes small group interactions and meaning construction in a social psychological context. He is noted for his approach called dramaturgy which analogizes people as actors who create performances in certain settings to manage their impressions to others in the "audience". Much of his work was drawn from classical sociologists George Herbert Mead and his work on the self (in Goffman's case, the "acting" self), and Emile Durkheim and his explorations of how rituals are enacted in people's daily lives.

Goffman's contributions to sociology are substantial and his work on *Asylums* (1961) is no exception. For this book, Goffman completed a field study in a mental health hospital in Washington, D.C. The lengthy subtitle for the book is *Essays on the Condition of the Social Situation of Mental Patients and Other Inmates* explaining that the work is primarily focused on mental patients, however, other "inmates" are examined in a supporting role. For this study, Goffman went undercover, posing as a recreation assistant to observe life on the inside of a mental institution.

The work is basically four essays, the first being a discussion on what Goffman termed 'total institutions'. These are explained as programs with certain characteristics, to differing degrees:

- all activities take place in the same location in the same format
- programs are directed by a single authority
- this activity is carried out with other institutionalized persons
- the activities are tightly scheduled and monitored
- the activities are carried out by both staff and inmates for a specified purpose (Goffman, 1961).

Examples of total institutions are prisons, military boot camps, convents and, of course, hospitals for mental patients and addicted people. There are many aspects to the inner workings of total institutions such as daily rituals, inmate culture, the ceremonial aspects of inmate activities, and experience of institutional staff. This chapter provides a comprehensive way of viewing organizations and it also lays the foundation for an examination of the total institutions formerly known as asylums.

The analysis of mental institutions begins with what Goffman refers to as the moral career of patients of mental institutions. Here he does not refer to career in the same sense as an occupational career, but rather the process that patients encounter—the pre-patient phase that occurs when people leave their homes to enter this new world, realizing their abandonment by the outside one; the inpatient phase where the people become fully indoctrinated to institutional life, and the ex-patient phase when people are discharged and return to society. All phases of this moral career affect the understanding of themselves and the selves of others in the system.

Goffman then provides an in-depth description of what he terms the underlife of the hospital. Describing not only the interactions that exist between patients, patients and staff, and patients and the institution itself, distinctions are made between the primary and secondary adjustments of mental patients. Primary adjustments refer to the reactions that are intentional and expected of an inmate, or the normal course of planned affairs. Secondary adjustments are those changes that are made to institutional life that "go around" the normal institutional dictates.

The final chapter entitled "The Medical Model and Mental Hospitalization: Some Notes on the Vicissitudes of the Tinkering Trades" is the most substantive for our examination. The type of model that is used in hospital setting generally, and in mental health hospitals specifically, is the personal-service occupational model in which there are clients, who have some need of repair, and there are servers, who have the training and tools to make the repair. The metaphor of a disabled car is provided—the client owns the car but is unable to fix the malfunction in the engine, therefore the owner finds a server (a mechanic) to repair it. A person who has a malfunction in the mental apparatus must also seek a server (a therapist) to repair that problem. The work setting is also important—current society has adopted a "workshop model" in which the repair work is made at the server's place of business (in the car example—a garage, and in the mental patient example—the asylum). In the asylums and in clinics, mental health practitioners are in the "tinkering trade", the very intrusive examinations that require explorations of both body and mind.

Goffman noted the client-server relationship in the workshop model currently used is not a good fit, however. It is ineffective as there are many more clients than servers, who do little in the way of repair. The very questions about maladjustment are not concrete as in normal client-server situations. People are labeled mentally ill and even provided with categories of malfunction (diagnoses), but as Thomas Szasz later noted, the idea of mental illness is socially constructed (we will get to this idea soon). People are hospitalized because they committed some behavior deemed abnormal: is this mental illness, then, or deviance? And are people treated or punished? In additions to the diagnostic problems in the current model, there are also treatment issues—for example, group therapy is used primarily in asylums as they are the only functional modality for so many clients (who, by the way, have different types of problems).

Goffman provided a brilliant analysis of mental health hospitalization but admittedly offered no solutions. He noted that if all mental institutions were emptied and closed, there would be new ones that would be demanded by relatives, the courts, and law enforcement. Interestingly, when deinstitutionalization of most of the mental institutions did occur, alternate forms of treatment in the form of community mental health formats were provided. Ending the book in his analysis of the personal-service occupational model, Goffman noted "mental patients can find themselves crushed by the weight of a service ideal that eases life for the rest of us" (1961, p. 386). The book, despite the intricate analysis of life in this type of total institution should be required reading for all people who work in a mental hospital setting—especially those in administration.

WHO IS MAD? AND WHO DECIDES?

Mental illness comes with a significant label, in fact, "madness" itself is a derogatory label today. It was the idea of labeling that concerned a group leading the "anti-psychiatry movement", beginning in the 1960s, though the seeds of this movement were planted years earlier. The antipsychiatry group was quite large and consisted of psychiatrists Thomas Szasz and R.D. Laing, sociologist Thomas Scheff, psychologist D.L. Rosenhan and others. Erving Goffman has often been placed in this camp as well, but his work on mental institutions was less an attack on established psychiatry than an observation of the mental health system. Even Michel Foucault is sometimes included in this group though he would have likely protested this label. The movement was placed against the backdrop of a zeitgeist that focused a critical eye on many areas of society, including the mental health system, which was deemed in need of repair. Even novels such as Ken Kersey's *One Flew Over the Cuckoo's Nest*, published in 1962 and made into a movie of the same name in 1975 brought to the lay audience an unflattering depiction of the mental health system (LaBruzza, 1997). In an era of questioning established social norms, the 1960s and 1970s left their mark on the field of mental health.

Thomas Szasz

Perhaps the best-known opponent of contemporary psychiatric diagnosis and practice was Thomas Szasz, a psychiatrist who wrote a series of books spanning decades and whose primary purpose was exposing the current mental health system as being fraudulent and deceptive. His corpus of work in this area began with a journal article entitled "The Myth of Mental Illness: Foundations of a Theory of Personal Conduct", originally published in 1960 in an academic journal and, carrying the same title, in book form in 1961. Szasz's thesis, which was met with shock in the psychiatric community and bemusement by the public, is that mental illness is not actually a disease in the medical sense and therefore has no business in the medical field. Mental illness is, in fact, a metaphor for disease rather than true disease. Mental illness is connected to the medical model for several reasons not related to any dictates of traditional medicine, and the consequences to society are such that a paradigm shift must be instituted for this reason.

According to Szasz (1961), mental illness was "invented" by the new field of psychiatry as control over people who deviated from social norms was passed from the religious institution to the eager and waiting hands of medicine. Physicians should as Benjamin Rush, Baron Richard von Krafft-Ebing, Jean-Martin Charcot, Pierre Janet, Sigmund Freud, and others promoted the idea of mental illness as a disease. With the backing of the major medical establishments, psychiatrists fortified their idea so successfully that it has become engrained in the culture of psychotherapy.

Szasz contended that people needing psychological treatment often do not seek it out willingly, but have it forced upon them by others, such as family, police, the courts, therefore mental health treatment is often coercive. For this reason, he called out psychiatry's lack of ethics. Szasz was concerned with the philosophical and moral rationale for forcing people to comply with medical treatment as normally treatment is voluntary.

The field of medicine, until the mid-nineteenth century, conceived of illness as a condition directly associated with the body and manifest as a deviation of the normal physical structure of the body. Physical assessments were developed to identify healthy organs and systems from unhealthy ones—aided by information from postmortem examinations. The medical field focused on bodily manifestations, not behavioral ones, to determine illness vs. non-illness. This is not to say that changes in body structure, such as a brain tumor, do not have behavioral manifestations but, according to Szasz, conditions such as this should be considered physical, not mental illnesses. Therefore, problems that have an environmental origin are not illnesses but metaphors of illness. Consider gambling, which is now included as a mental disorder in the DSM-5—is this a brain disorder? If so, what scientific evidence supports this claim? Does a person who has never been around gambling activity have this disorder? If in the future we can establish a link with the brain, it should be reclassified as a physical disorder and people with this genetic problem will do well to avoid casinos. Hopefully, this illustrates Szasz's point about the problems in classifying disorders.

Szasz (1961) reached into sociology and social psychology when he described behavior on the part of patients as communication, where game playing attempts to cope with an internal crisis. The early mental health classification of "hysteria" is instructive here. Hysteria was an early catch-all phase for some general instability and was often linked to malingering, or the faking of illness. This diagnosis no longer officially exists but perhaps, as Szasz posited, is an issue involving communication—the patients are trying to communicate something if therapists are attuned to their needs.

Szasz believed that people, including mental patients, should be considered autonomous beings and should not have their rights curtained by an overcontrolling system that purports to be a medical institution. The libertarian ideological strain in this work is evident here. His idea that those behaviors that have been mistakenly labeled mental illness should be termed "problems in living" and treated in a non-medical fashion that does not deprive them of their liberties (Szasz, 1961). Think of the medical interventions of the past century such as lobotomies and shock treatments and how that fits into his analysis.

R.D. Laing

R.D. Laing was another prominent writer in the anti-psychiatry movement. While Szasz attacked the psychiatric establishment using the metaphor of the mental illness as myth, Laing provided his critique of psychiatry using a philosophical approach to explain the world of the schizoid patient in his most prominent work, 1960's *A Divided Self: An Existential Study of Sanity and Madness* (Laing, 1960), which contained his ideas introduced in a journal the previous year.

Laing was a Scottish psychiatrist who, like many others during the period, was trained in psychoanalysis. He was born into a family with material comforts but little love or concern; his relationship with his mother was particularly conflictual. His academic background was very broad and, in addition to psychiatry and psychology, his interests included philosophy, literature, and theology: this broad background would inform his desire to move psychiatry into new areas. He was working in a mental institution during the 1950s when he decided to try an informal experiment in which he had the hospital staff remain calm despite the patients' emotional outbursts; this experiment resulted in the quelling of antagonisms without the use of drugs, electric shocks, or physical restraints. The experiment reinforced his ideas that the human connection with the hospital workers was the most important thing in returning patients to a level which would assist in their treatment. His goal was to convince his colleagues—very big names in the field at the time such as W.D.R. Fairburn, Donald Winnicott, John Bowlby, and Melanie Klein, that his philosophical approach to psychiatry, known as "existential phenomenology", would provide an effective and novel change to the treatment of the mentally ill (Laing, 1994) by focusing on the world view of the patients from a non-judgmental stance.

In *Self,* Laing used the existential phenomenological perspective to explain how his schizoid patients were basically trapped in a world not understood by many in the mental health profession. And psychiatry, he claimed, had little desire to develop that understanding of the mental patient's pain, preferring to focus on medicalizing it and keeping a safe distance from that pain. Mental health practitioners saw mentally ill people as objects rather than people. Laing's interest was primarily in understanding the world of schizophrenic patients and he posited that psychotic patients experienced the split in two ways—externally, with society, and internally, within themselves. The psychotic patient, Laing surmised, loses a basic sense of autonomy and therefore the patient's sense of connection with the world is disturbed. The patient becomes unembodied and in contrast to the mentally healthy "embodied" person, who is alive and connected to the world, feels unsubstantial and frustrated. The desire of the schizoid patient is to preserve selfhood and when this does not occur, the existence of a false self appears. With the appearance of this false self, odd and eccentric behavior occurs (Laing, 1960).

Laing felt a psychotic person's early life is important and efforts should be taken by mental health personnel to develop a comprehensive psychosocial examination and continue to follow up on those observations. He acknowledged this is a difficult task as the person's break from reality can be substantial, but this is a task that must be achieved to understand a psychotic person's inner experience. Laing believed the field of psychiatry was not adequately performing this task, favoring the comfortable, traditional medical model for patients. He noted that people do not *catch* schizophrenia in the same way people catch colds—they *have* the disorder. And how they act in the world is related to how they are treated by the profession, as Laing states, "What the schizophrenic is to us determines very considerably what we are to him, and hence his actions" (Laing, 1960, p.34). While *Self* was not a direct challenge to the field of psychiatry as some of the other works we have discussed in this chapter, his subsequent writings would take a more confrontational tone. This work, the first of several by a then 28-year-old psychiatrist, provided a more philosophical element to the antipsychiatry movement.

Although trained in psychiatry, Laing made significant contributions to sociology, to the point of developing his own version of the "sociological imagination"; the field, however, has been slow in acknowledging his contributions (Scott & Thorpe, 2006). Most obvious is his emphasis on the social environment rather than the ideas of biological determinism and biological reductionism (the idea that biology determines eventual outcomes and that thoughts and behaviors can be reduced to this level) that had taken over psychiatry in the wake of Freudianism's descent. His focus on the self, albeit in a disordered way, further develops the work of G.H. Mead. His attempts to understand the world view of psychotic patients makes use of another sociological concept called 'subjective understanding', developed by sociologist Max Weber. In addition, Laing's focus on oppressive institutional structures and the labeling of the mentally ill is a contribution to the sociology of deviance. In many ways, Laing's work compliments Szasz's problems in living model (Scott & Thorpe, 2006).

D.L. Rosenhan

Another reinforcement to the idea of mental illness as a social construction was developed from a research study published in a famous article entitled "On Being Sane in Insane Places" (1973) by D.L. Rosenhan. This article received an enormous amount of attention as the author, a psychologist, concluded there is little difference between sanity and insanity, at least as far as can be determined even by trained mental health practitioners. The study involved participants who were not mentally ill that were admitted into various psychiatric hospitals pretending to hear voices. These "pseudopatients", after admittance, were instructed to act normally and just observe and take notes. The staff at the institutions did not seem to notice they were, in fact, sane and created ways to justify their "illness". Some of the hospital inmates noticed something was amiss, however.

In a follow-up study (basically a control group study), staff were advised there would be people entering their hospitals who were posing as mental patients who were not actually ill; several of the patients were picked as being those who were mentally ill, however, at this study, no actual pseudopatients were used. Rosenhan concluded that mental health diagnoses and labels are extremely tenuous, especially if the trained practitioners cannot tell the "sane" from the "insane". The setting—the hospital—was an environment that was expected to house the mentally ill; alternatively, when it was believed that pseudopatients were in their midst, they were looking for, and found, fakers, even though they didn't exist (Rosenhan, 1973).

Thomas Scheff

Thomas Scheff is a sociologist who described a labeling process that occurs in the mental health field that defines mental illness as a form of deviance in his work *Being Mentally Ill: A Sociological Theory* (1999, originally published in 1966). Conditions that are conceived of as psychological symptoms are actually forms of rule-breaking. He specifically referred to "residential rule-breaking" to define acts that do not have a socially recognized form of deviance. It is the social construction of the activity that defines it as mental illness rather than psychological conditions normally associated with it.

In a later edition of *Being Mentally Ill*, Scheff (1999) expressed a need for the mental health field to adopt an interdisciplinary approach which includes recent advances in bio-psychiatry. However, he maintains that to dismiss labeling theory from this approach is "premature" (Scheff, 1999, p. xiii). A defining characteristic of the labeling approach is the focus on the stigma that comes from being mentally ill, a topic that will be discussed in chapter eight.

AGAINST THE ANTIPSYCHIATRY MOVEMENT

Although the antipsychiatry movement shook up the field of mental health, many never bought into the idea that mental health diagnosis and treatment are socially constructed and ambiguous; they also rejected the critical analysis that has for decades taunted the mental health field. We will look at some of the charges leveled at psychiatry including the idea that mental illness does not fit in the medical model (particularly the issue of disease-in-the-body vs. disease-in-the-mind), that mental illness is but a myth or a misleading label, and that diagnostic categories are inappropriate in evaluating mental illness, and the idea of historical accuracy of the claims of critics.

The argument that mental illness doesn't neatly fit into the medical model is a noteworthy point. However, many mental disorders do have a somatic component and the physical and mental activity work in tandem. As psychotherapy services move from psychiatrists to non-medical therapists such as psychologists, social workers, marriage and family therapists, and professional counselors, this doesn't seem to be as much of an issue as it was decades ago when the antipsychiatry movement was at its zenith. A symbiotic relationship between the two fields has produced many benefits to patients.

The medical model was perceived by the antipsychiatrists as inappropriate for mental health issues, primarily because of the body-mind contradiction—the idea that diseases of the body are not analogous to disturbances of the mind. Some psychiatric scholars (Roth & Kroll, 1986) have had trouble understanding why psychiatry would not be considered in the same vein as other medical specialties. According to these scholars, there are certainly more similarities than differences, such as identical "goals, methods, subject matter, ethics, and responsibilities" (Roth & Kroll, 1986, p. 58). The scholars also note the term "biopsychosocial model" might be a more appropriate term as it encompasses psychological and social factors, not only biological ones. The medical field addresses more than just "lumps, lesions, and germs" (Roth & Kroll, 1986, p. 13) and there are many environmental concerns that contribute to and are affected by physical conditions—the field of public health which consists of organized efforts to address environmental conditions in communities that affect the health of its citizens—is an example of how a biopsychosocial approach can be beneficial.

The idea of mental illness being a *myth* has been questioned. The American Heritage Dictionary of the English Language (2000) defines "myth" as a "fictitious story, person, or thing" (p. 1164). An elaboration of this definition from the dictionary is "a popular belief or story that has become associated with a person, institution, or occurrence, especially one that is considered to illustrate a cultural ideal" (AHDEL, 2000, p.1164). Using the initial definition, it is difficult to see how mental disorders are fictitious, because their significance is too real to be inconsequential, however, the use of the second definition—that mental illness is a cultural narrative—is somewhat easier to accept. If mental illness is viewed in its historical context as an unfolding story, the fluid nature of our understandings suggests that a social constructionist perspective is plausible. It has been suggested that instead of the term myth, "metaphor" is a more apt description of mental illness. Defined as "one thing conceived as representing another; a symbol" (AHDEL, 2000, p.1104), a metaphor approach indicates that mental illness represents physical health; this is obvious, but whether it *should* represent physical health is the question. Even though this illustrates the role of semantics, the use of the term myth in describing mental illness has certainly been problematic.

Diagnostic categories were considered by those in the antipsychiatry camp as social constructions which were arbitrary and potentially stigmatizing. However, the idea of categorizing things is a natural one and has an evolutionary function (Roth & Kroll, 1986). Even single cell organisms such as amoeba can differentiate between things that are food and things that are dangerous to their existence. The eons that medicine has existed culminated in a long effort of classifying diseases and disorders to better treat them, successively building on knowledge; to consider the classification systems that have developed over this time as either useless or as having ulterior motives can be perceived as counterproductive. One scholar (Spitzer, 1975) noted that the terms used in Rosenhan's study— "sane" and "insane"—are not diagnostic categories, but even using this language, the psychiatrists involved in this experiment were responding to the patients' complaints when they admitted them; based on the available information the diagnosis of schizophrenia was correct, not taking this information and formulating a diagnosis would not be providing appropriate patient care. Weiner (1975) stated the hypothesis used in the Rosenhan study—that trained professionals are unable to detect pseudopatients from real patients—is wrong and claimed that if an experiment was conducted that placed 20 pseudopatients and 20 real patients in a hospital setting, the differences would be easily detected by trained diagnosticians. To add to this conversation Crown (1975) stated the type of "stooge research" as used in the Rosenhan study provided inadequate data and could be considered unethical.

The historical background provided by some of the people in the movement, particularly Foucault, has been severely challenged. For example, the idea of the "ship of fools" creates some very vivid imagery about the early days of treatment of the mentally ill, but it has little basis in fact. Kushner (1998) claims the antipsychiatrists accepted Foucault's premises, even with historical inaccuracies and lack of knowledge of mental health practice, fitting their ideas in with his historical fiction while not realizing his claims which have come under such scrutiny fuels the scientific method by being subject to investigation and testing contradictory findings. Perhaps social constructionism can assist science in this matter.

Johnson (1990), while agreeing the labeling process described as sociologists Goffman and Scheff provides "uncomfortable insights" (p. 61), patients with mental illness do have major psychological issues that must be addressed therapeutically, even though the process of labeling has occurred. In other words, the social phenomenon of labeling and the existence of mental illness both represent reality.

Also, while accepting the importance of the anti-psychiatry social constructionists, Horowitz (2002) describes some limitations of the constructionist approach. While cultural situations do create how mental health diagnosis and treatment are constructed and provide one explanation for mental illness, concrete biological explanations are generally more accepted in Western societies. If the main criteria for mental illness is based on culture, there are many limitations in comparison with other disordered conditions—the lack of conceived standards that function as a point of reference promotes further ambiguity in understanding different forms of mental illness, inside cultures or among them. Additionally, the social constructionist approach conflicts with diagnostic psychology in that it does account for the differing levels of severity of functions between the various conditions deemed mental illness.

REFLECTIONS ON THE MOVEMENT

Even though the influence of the antipsychiatry movement waned in the 1970s and 1980s, being replaced by advances in neurobiology and psychotherapy techniques, in some countries provisions of the movement were continued. The movement was carried out to its extreme in the mid- and late 1970s as leftist Italian psychiatrists lead by Franco Basaglia sought to use the antipsychiatry movement to change the structure of the country's mental health system by using these tactics:

- asylums were closed and replaced with community programs
- compulsory commitments were outlawed
- restraints, seclusion, and invasive procedures were ended
- psychological and psychopharmacological interventions were rejected

The program, called Psichiatria Democratica, however, was not monitored scientifically and eventually became a political rather than a social movement: it even proved to be an impediment to progressive change as it continued (Berlim, Fleck, & Shorter, 2003).

The 1990s were dubbed the "Decade of the Brain", with the brain being the first bodily organ to be provided a decade (Sherman, 2001). Funds were provided for research in this area and this focus preempted earlier ideas about finding the causes and treatment in the social environment and focused more on finding the causes in the body, or "not in our minds but in our brains" (Sherman, 2001, p. 96). Suddenly, a belief in scientific advancement, coupled with the lure of huge financial gains from drugs to treat these brain disorders returned psychiatry to its former medical roots.

However, it can be said that the antipsychiatry movement had some positive effects on the field. It might be insightful to look at the movement as having provided us with some information on issues of relevance today. It is questionable that the system currently operates in an organized effort to keep many people in an oppressed condition. This argument was more salient prior to the deinstitutionalization efforts which disbursed many patients from hospitals into outpatient programs, but creating an environment that thwarts abuses of power should always be a major objective in mental health programs. It is likely that the newer forms of psychotherapy which involve collaboration by patient and therapist are a preventative factor in this regard.

The labeling issue is one that needs continued scrutiny as the stigma that exists in mental health must be addressed before positive change can occur. Another area that is felt that should be seriously reconsidered is the issue of mental health diagnosis. A diagnostic guide is necessary for a professional field to provide adequate services for its clients and it must acknowledge new information as it becomes available through new research. However, the fact that more and more aspects of normal human existence are considered mental illnesses should be a concern that perhaps that everyday life is becoming medicalized, as Thomas Szasz claimed.

A new movement?

It could be said that the movement did not end, it simply morphed into what has become an attack on psychopharmacology and the DSM. One of the most vocal critics, Allen Frances, states that "diagnostic inflation" and over-medication are the problems currently plaguing psychiatry (Frances, 2013). Francis, who was on the panel for the DSM-IV and the DSM-5, strongly criticizes the current (and perhaps future) diagnostic manual for overextending its reach into everyday problems that do not need to be categorized as mental disorders. He also notes how pharmaceutical companies (Big Pharma) are targeting these "new" disorders with a host of drugs that, rather than contributing to a cessation of the problem, creates new ones in its place, such as addiction. Frances (2013) points out, however, that his concerns in these areas (which are significant), do not connote "antipsychiatry" as he is not against the profession, just the current changes in the areas listed.

Many other voices have recently been raised in the criticisms in mental health diagnostics and psychopharmacology—these voices can be in found in publications by not only psychiatrists and other practitioners of the mental health field, but also academics, and investigative journalists, among others, including medical historians such as Edward Shorter. All of these decry the use of diagnostic inflation and the improper use of many pharmacological alternatives to psychotherapy.

Medical journalist Robert Whitaker (2015), describes an "epidemic" of psychiatric medications that are not helping but rather contributing to many mental health and physical health problems. From the release of Thorazine in the 1950s, and more recently anti-anxiety medications, antidepressants, and Lithium for bipolar disorder, these "magic bullets" are making society sicker. While acknowledging the role of social factors in the increase in the incidence of mental illness, the author states that many of the current conditions are iatrogenic, which means created by the mental health care system itself. Whitaker (2015) posits the expansion of diagnostic categories for both adults and children and subsequent medication of these patients is to blame for the epidemic.

Another journalist, Ethan Watters (2011) adopts a cross cultural approach to the mental health field and observes the role that globalization plays in formulating belief systems about mental illness. In American society, the response to national emergencies has been to move quickly to create new forms of illness followed by new medications to "fix" the problems. An analogy is made to relief efforts to provide sick natives with blankets "without considering the pathogens that hide deep in the fabric" (Watters, 2011, p.253). Drawing from Shorter (1992), the author describes how cultures create "symptom pools" in which to place the effects of stressors of different collective crises. The Western model of DSM diagnosis followed by massive medication dumps is a characteristic that has been exported around the globe. Watters questions if this approach is desirable.

Kirk, Gomory, and Cohen (2013), social work scholars, explain how psychiatry, which is touted as the science of madness, is itself mad in that it is supported by flimsy research, research that is directly tied into money that benefits not only Big Pharma but also Big Government. Extending the work of Szasz, the authors describe the coercive process that continues to exist, even in today's community-based settings. Mental health treatment, especially in the form of psychopharmacology, the authors claim, uses the guise of "mental illness as a brain disorder" to coerce consumers to buy into this "mad science", through use of coercion that has been effective.

CONCLUSION

A sociological perspective on mental health has the value of allowing us the ability to step back and see the connection between individual troubles and social issues, using an intellectual tool known as the sociological imagination to view mental illness through both biography and history, allowing a more comprehensive understanding of mental illness, mental health, and the mental health system.

Many scholars have provided a sociological vantage point to the mental health field, but not all of these were professional sociologists. This theorizing took place during a certain point in time—the mid to later twentieth century—a time when many changes were taking place not only in the field but also in society generally. A questioning of norms and social institutions took on an antiestablishment zeitgeist both inside the mental health establishment and in the greater society. Erich Fromm, Michel Foucault, Erving Goffman, Thomas Szasz, R.D. Laing, D.L. Rosenhan, and Thomas Scheff questioned the features of psychotherapy, psychopharmacology, and institutional and professional practices (deemed violations of civil rights) and all, to different degrees, have been classified as a group known as the anti-psychiatrists, though most rejected the label.

As the major force in psychiatry waned, a new approach has entered the field as ideas about biological causes and treatments have come to the fore, returning psychiatry to its roots reinforcing medical treatments, including psychopharmacology. Another group of mental health scholars, practitioners, and writers have once again emerged (in a similar vein as the anti-psychiatrists) that have rejected certain components of modern psychiatry, primarily the diagnostic process, mentioned in the last chapter, and the extensive use of chemical interventions to treat emotional issues.

The field of mental health has primarily been under the watchful eyes of psychiatry and psychology. However, sociology offers a different approach in that it focuses on the social environment contributes to mental health. They also observe the social responses and the institutions that have developed due to poor mental health in society. A sociological perspective often challenges the dominant outlook and the taken-for-granted ways of seeing the world. American democracy has provided a substructure that allows different vantage points which allow for changes in the social structure where changes are needed, including the field of psychotherapy.

Chapter 6

A SYSTEMS APPROACH TO THE MENTAL HEALTH SYSTEM

> "Human beings are as much engaged in using social systems as in being used by them. Men are social systems-using and social systems-building creatures."
>
> (Alvin Gouldner 1970, p. 220)

AN UNDERSTANDING OF SYSTEMS

We understand the complex web of mental health-related organizations as a system, but what exactly does that mean? What type of system is it? What are its parts? In what ways does it function appropriately? In what ways does it function inadequately? What are the consequences of its functioning appropriately or inadequately? To answer these questions, we must learn a little about social systems theory.

The term system is associated with many things. We normally think of the systems existing in the natural world such as solar, weather, and water systems; however, they also exist in the social world in the form of family, political, economic, and religious systems, as well as numerous others. While the animal societies of the natural world operate in a highly functional, well-coordinated manner based on genetic predisposition, human societies, in contrast, operate in highly individualistic, egoistic (or self-serving) ways but must have some level of utilitarianism (consisting of actions for the best interest of the whole) to remain in existence (Nolan & Lenski, 2011).

Systems can be defined simply as entities that possess interrelated components which have been described as "bundles of relations" (Rapaport, 1968). This description reflects the current practice that today of "bundling" items to be purchased together (such as books, internet services, or insurance policies) with the understanding that these things have something in common that, when included together, constitute a more complete and desirable package.

Systems can be defined by the following characteristics:

- they exist as whole separate entities with discernable boundaries
- the entities are comprised of parts or elements that interact and have a consistent (rather than random) organizational structure
- there is an objective or function it seeks to fulfil, which requires a degree of stability and a means of controlling these functions to achieve the goal (Stewart, Winborn, Burks, Johnson, & Engelkes, 1978).

There are many terms and concepts related to systems theory such as *equilibrium, feedback, interdependence, energy, dynamics, evolution, structure, function, action, transaction, complexity,* and *boundaries.* Other terms that describe the operation of systems include *dominance* and *hierarchy,* as all parts of systems are not equal, nor are all systems equal. Other terms include *organismic,* which is a term that reflects the organ analogy in systems thinking, and *cybernetics,* which refers to the communication processes that exist through automatic control within systems. Communication is an important concept as well as it creates the transfer of energy that allows the system to change and accomplish its goals (Anderson & Carter, 1990). Information exchange through the various parts of the system and subsystems is referred to as feedback. Feedback, positive and negative, is the response to activity which allows systems to self-direct, adapt, and seek its goals; it involves "not only the echo but the adjustment made to the echo" (Anderson & Carter, 1990, p.37). As societies evolve, subsystems are created to appropriately deal with the changes brought about by changes in social norms. The systems perspective has many branches and basically posits that people in society, as living beings must behave in certain ways that promote functionality for the whole (Churchman, 1979).

The mental health system as viewed from the systems perspective, for example, includes the physical structures (hospitals, clinics and other locales, such as schools where counseling is provided); the mental health personnel (practitioners, support staff, and all associated workers); the apparatus for payment of services (which include insurance, private pay, Medicare, Medicaid); the various programs (in-patient, out-patient, 12 step programs) and methods of service provision (individual, family, group, couple), and methodology (cognitive-behavioral, psychodynamic, brief short term, narrative).

EARLY FORMULATIONS OF SOCIETY AS A SYSTEM

Some early social philosophers such as Herbert Spencer viewed society as a system of interrelated parts that function much like a machine. This orgiastic approach is comprised of social institutions such as the government, economy, family, education, and religion and these parts are interdependent upon each other. Another analogy with the orgiastic approach is the human body—the parts of the body have certain functions and when these parts adequately provide their purposes, the body is viewed as "healthy". When the institutions of the social body are working correctly, society is also perceived as being in good functional shape—a healthy society. Spencer's orgiastic approach has certain key features:

- it is applicable to human systems; the whole of the object is more than the sum of its parts
- the whole creates the defining characteristic of the parts; the parts can only be understood as components of the whole
- the parts are interdependent upon each other (Phillips, 1970).

Spencer viewed the parts in the natural world as providing functions for the whole; in the social world it is reversed and the whole provides for its components (Olson, 1970). It was Emile Durkheim who saw a collective conscience (shared social values and morals) as the means to keep these parts functioning in a cohesive fashion, keeping society healthy (Salerno, 2004).

Influenced by Spencer, sociologists would later analogize systems that exist in the social world with those in the natural environment. Lester Frank Ward was an early American sociologist who drew from his background as a botanist to observe the social world in a similar manner as the natural one. Ward saw the evolution of society as passing from genetic (natural) and telic (synthetic or social) structures and functions. Society evolves, according to Ward, in a "symbodal" model rather than a linear one—by this he envisioned social development through a series of branches that emanate from the trunk and to form their own type of government (Scott, 1976).

Similarly, Robert Park also adopted the ecological approach and dubbed it "human ecology". Using the plant world as an analogy, Park examined such concepts as invasion, succession, and dominance as they relate to interpersonal relations between people. Park, colleague Earnest Burgess, and others that constitute the group of theorists known as the Chicago School of sociology, examined their rapidly changing city as an ecological system, rooted in nature ("human nature") and divided by natural areas that made up the character of the urban environment. Due to the changes in structure that occurred from demographic fluctuations, "social patterns were etched in space" (Goldfield & Brownell, 1979).

Following in this analogy of social systems was the work of sociologist Talcott Parsons, who further developed this orgiastic model into a theoretical approach called structural functionalism. Parsons paid notice to how systems are structured and how the functioning of the various parts of the system allows them to perform their purposes. He also noted their ability to effectively work with the other parts of the system to benefit the whole. His structural functionalist approach examined systems and their subsystems from four levels:

1. The organism
2. The personal
3. The social structure
4. The cultural (Parsons, 1951)

Good mental health is functional at the organism level because a system evolves appropriately when the subsystem parts are healthy; it is functional at the personal level as good mental health results is a better life; it is functional at the structural level because better mental health results in a stronger and government and an enhanced family life; at the cultural level it reveals national concerns over the functioning of society (Levin, 1991) and the measures taken to advocate for those who have mental disorders.

In his description of Parsons' systems theory, Gouldner explains his ideas of how systems evolve and differentiate (or separate): "social systems are born as living organisms, but everywhere they are becoming machines" (Gouldner 1970, p. 210). Technology can cause problems as we progress through the process of culture lag, as our technological ability sometimes outpaces our social values. The effects of this differentiation process which is like the rationalization process, where increasing levels of calculation and measurement are sought to promote advancement and predictable efficiency. The machine analogy is an interesting one as humans have been concerned about the growing use of machines and possible consequences resulting from their ascendance in human affairs. Indeed, this concern has been metaphorically described by a sociologist at mid-twentieth century as a machine (in this case, a spacecraft) which has dropped its pilot, flying off wildly into space (Horkheimer, 1947). Numerous cautionary tales evoke this concern. However, it is possible, as some early sociologists believe that technology contains the seeds that allow us to progress. Perhaps technology that is carefully monitored provides the greatest hope, and this applies to the mental health system as well.

A notable adjunct to systems models was provided by mathematician Norbert Wiener and anthropologist Gregory Bateson in the form of cybernetics. Wiener sought to find common elements between incongruent systems such as human nervous systems and machine operations; he looked for these commonalities in the form of communication processes and control measures. These "first order" cybernetics were further developed by later scholars as "second order cybernetics" (or "cybernetics of cybernetics"), an understanding that any observation of systems requires an observer, who as part of the system cannot make interpretations without prejudice. This would later lead to the theoretical position known as social constructionism in which perspectives of reality are governed by the often-flawed position of the observer (Drack & Pouvreau, 2015)—the reader will think back to the previous chapter in which the concept of mental illness itself was questioned by the "anti-psychiatrists".

Although many early formulations about systems focused on equilibrium, cohesion, and interdependence, we should not ignore the role of tension that develops between systems. As systems advance, they often develop in ways that do not coalesce, or do so in different directions (Timascheff, 1967). The case of the criminalization of mental illness reflects this idea—when the criminal justice system develops and expands ideas into what constitutes "deviant" behavior, conflicts arise between the mental health and criminal justice systems. The idea of the criminalization of mental illness is explored in more detail in chapter eight

General Systems Theory

To provide a comprehensive examination of mental-health-as-a-system, it could be beneficial to turn back to some of the earliest ideas on the systems perspective. One of the earliest systematic formulations to be applied to social systems was created by an Austrian botanist named Ludwig von Bertalanffy, beginning in the 1920s and developing into a seminal theoretical framework known as general systems theory (or sometimes the singular general *system* theory) for understanding human life as it relates to systems. Its importance in understanding the system of mental health is so significant that it deserves exploration on the topic as a broadly encompassing model. Bertalanffy's analysis of systems extended from biology and the other national sciences into the social sciences of sociology, anthropology, psychology and philosophy, as well as the applied fields of psychiatry, engineering, and systems analysis. Therefore, general systems theory observes systems from the microscopic levels of cells to complex macro level cultural arrangements in large societies. The approach is consequently interdisciplinary and integrative and by necessity requires a grand theoretical scheme.

Bertalanffy (1968) specifically addressed systems as applied to psychology and psychiatry, complaining that early psychology envisioned humans as robots. The use of a systems approach, he assumed, provided a better examination of the human psyche than behaviorism, psychoanalysis, or cybernetic models by seeing humans as "an active personality system" (Bertalanffy, 1968 p. 207) which utilizes symbols to appropriately function in the environment. Bertalanffy believed Talcott Parson's work involved an overemphasis on the maintenance of stability, equilibrium, and homeostasis and ignored the role of conflict and change. Likewise, mental disorders develop when a conflict exists between the individual and culture. It is through the lens of culture that psychopathology is created. In Bertalanffy's view, psychology and psychiatry must incorporate the role of culture, as a system, to correctly address mental illness; this is consistent with the notion of symptom pools and culture-bound symptoms that will be discussed soon.

Other Systems Models

Another model that might be important in understanding a systems approach is one proposed by Uri Bronfenbrenner; this model based on what is sometimes called the "human ecology theory", or bioecological theory, which Bronfenbrenner developed over many years. This theoretical approach is one of the most famous frameworks for understanding human development in society, influencing policy for global organizations such as the World Health Organization (WHO) and United Nations Children's Fund (UNICEF) (Velez-Agosto, Soto-Crespo, Vizcarrondo-Oppenheim, Vega-Molina, & Garcia, 2017). Bronfenbrenner (1977)'s model is illustrated in a series of concentric circles that circle the core:

- the center is the microsystem, which consists of the immediate systems in which the person is involved (Bronfenbrenner focused on child psychology so the family and the educational, day care, and religious institutions form this system)
- the mesosystem which consists of a linkage between two or more microsystems (such as the family and the school)
- the exosystem which consists of those agencies, institutions, and service providers that affect the individual less directly, but which do influence that person's life (such as various governmental agencies, informal social networks, and transportation systems)

- the macrosystem which refers to the customs and traditions of the culture which an individual is socialized (formal and information laws, beliefs, and rituals)—this level system of comprised of all the other systems.
- the chronosystem was added as the model advanced and reflects how the course of time affects the individual in the various systems; in effect, it takes into account changes in the individual's lifespan (Smith & Hamon, 2012).

While Bronfenbrenner's model is very useful in its conception of understanding systems, it is simplistic and rigid, therefore other schools of systems theory have sought to alter the model.

An update of Bronfenbrenner's conceptualization, called the "cultural microsystem model" (Velez-Agosto et al., 2017), has been developed and places culture as a central component throughout the various systems (self, home, neighborhood, educational programs, laws, social services, media, and chronos). Schematically, this scheme is represented in swirls and broken lines in lieu of rigidly divided concentric circles to represent a free flow of energy between systems. The chronos system is visualized as moving the other systems from one state to another as events in history change all systems, not just the cultural system (this is the "historical push and shove" mentioned by C. Wright Mills). Therefore, culture is a part of all systems—the schools, day care environments, etc.—and policy initiatives must consider the cultural aspects of systems at all levels.

SYSTEMS AT DIFFERENT LEVELS

In taking a systems approach, it is best to analyze the different systems that are operational, starting with the personal (or individual) system and extending outward through the family system, the community and neighborhood systems, the health care system, and the cultural system. Imagine these levels as emanating from the personal and extending through the other systems with concentric circles but with spaces in the circles that allow for the energy exchange that occurs across them.

The personal system

The human body is itself a container of a vast number of systems:

- the central nervous system
- endocrine system
- respiratory system

- reproductive system
- digestive system
- cognitive system
- circulatory system

And these, of course, are but a few of the many systems in the body. As mentioned earlier, these systems and their component parts must appropriately perform their individual functions for the personal system to be healthy. For purposes of our analysis, we will focus on the personality system and the process through which the self is developed.

People are socialized into the dictates of the greater society and they are expected to conform to the norms of society. Emile Durkheim referred to a collective conscience that created the cohesion and solidarity that sustains societies and protects them from a state called anomie, or lack of adequate integration of norms in society. However, an overabundance of social integration is unhealthy, and people simply become automatons, accepting all aspects of culture, including harmful ones.

There must be some degree of individuation, or individual growth that results from differentiation from the other parts of a system, in which people can explore ideas about the self. The term "self" is a commonly used one, but it has specific meanings about personhood. While the personality is often perceived of as a stable entity, reflecting characteristics in an individual's life that remain stable over the life span, the self is normally seen as a dynamic object that changes due to life circumstances and interactions with others. The sociological perspective known as symbolic interactionism stresses how this self is developed through "significant symbols", such as language, physical gestures, and signs in communication with others (Mead, 1934). We often use society as a mirror to develop views of ourselves based on the responses of others—a concept known as the "looking glass self" (Cooley, 1902). Similarly, psychiatrist Harry Stack Sullivan (1953) noted how the internalization of reflected appraisals by other people during developmental process contributes to the formation of the individual self.

As the individuation process continues, an identity is formed. In the case of mentally ill people, the identity is often perceived by many others to be a deviant identity. Labeling theorists of the symbolic interactionist school of sociology note how primary deviance occurs when an activity is deemed to be outside the norm. Secondary deviance occurs when the person performing the action is formally provided with an official label, such as a DSM diagnosis or an involuntary commitment to a mental hospital; when the person accepts that label, this creates a self-fulfilling prophecy that maintains the stigmatization (this, we should recall, was a primary concern of the scholars of the anti-psychiatry movement). There is a third type of deviance in this process—tertiary deviance, which assumes people do not always accept the deviant label on a subjective basis (Sandstrom, Lively, Martin, & Fine, 2014) and ignore the prophecy that foretells a deviant lifestyle—this is a primary goal for those who advocate for the mentally ill.

People are social creatures, greatly influenced by what they feel others think about them. Selves can be very fragile and there are many defensive mechanisms in play that are used to protect the vulnerable self; included in these mechanisms are:

- denial of unpleasant thoughts
- escapism
- repression of painful images
- internalization of problematic thoughts (Hamachek, 1978).

Attacks on the self can create emotional stress resulting in mental disorder; if the protective defenses fail to provide this function or if they become too extreme, this too can produce adverse mental conditions.

Psychologist Abraham Maslow (1943) created one of the world's most recognizable personal systems. Schematically, it is often represented as a triangle with different levels of human needs, starting here at the bottom:

- the basic physiological needs (food, clothing, and shelter)
- safety needs (security and protection)
- belonging and love needs (intimate social relationships)
- esteem needs (prestige and positive regard from peers)
- self-actualization (achieving personal ambitions and creative endeavors).

People must have their needs met at each stage to progress to the next. Good mental health is a result of adequate passage through these stages.

Families and small groups

Some approaches to understanding family life emphasize the types of behaviors and activity by the members that contribute to the stability or instability of family functioning. Others observe the conflict that is created between members, attend to the exchanges that are made between members, or analyze the external conditions that create disharmony. Some focus on the individual, others emphasize a mix of the social and biological, and others support philosophical or ideological positions. From a systems perspective, families are groupings that are highly interdependent and a change in one member affects the whole family system.

Families can be viewed as being open, random, or closed/enmeshed. In open families, members are bound by affective ties and possess open channels of communication where feedback is promoted. In random families, there is a significant lack of boundary and rule maintenance which causes the younger members to feel there is a lack of concern for them. In closed (or enmeshed) families, there is an overabundance of closeness which allows little room for individual group and the establishment of a separate self (Smith & Hamon, 2012).

Families are collections of personalities, or superpersonalities according to early American sociologist Earnest Burgess (1926) who devised a typology of two classifications of families: the integrated type which possesses appropriate levels of interdependence, discipline, and family rituals, and the unintegrated type that fails to provide functional role expectations for the family members (Smith & Hamon, 2012).

Family systems approaches also seek to find equilibrium, or the balance between order and change. Family traditions and shared values provide the order needed to deal with the stressors that come with the development of the individual families—stressors that occur as new members enter, grow, change, and eventually leave the family system. Due to the family being the primary agent of socialization, this is often where psychopathological symptoms begin. And if the pathology is genetic, it obviously has its origins in the family, and the dysfunctions will be maintained there unless outside intervention occurs. Family therapy is a field that focuses on how psychopathological symptoms that appear in one member of the family affects the others.

It was mentioned in chapter four that family therapy approaches normally adopt the systems model. Using our earlier description of systems, it is certainly easy to conceive of families as small social systems with component parts that coordinate in ways to accomplish some specific tasks including primarily socialization and social control. The family, after all, is a unit of the larger cultural system and is expected to function in ways that mirror society. (Anderson & Carter, 1990).

Small non-familial groups in therapy often possess characteristics like those of families, since both are small systems. Group treatment models also often use a systems conceptualization in their applications to various groupings of people with different needs—psychological or addiction related. Therapeutic models such as systematic counseling utilize a holistic approach that considers the various systems that exist in a person's environment (Stewart et al., 1978). Although group counseling originally was based on an individual treatment model, a systems model developed directly from general systems theory, and understands groups as living social systems that respond to therapeutic interventions in various ways and in which a change in the status of one member of the group will influence the others. In addition, since groups possess a self-regulating system of equilibrium maintenance (much like families), interventions will create a level of disharmony, resulting in anxiety. The anxiety must be affectively handled by the group leader to promote growth and change in the members (Donigan & Malnati, 1997).

Communities

Communities are collectivities that have distinct components:

- a collective identity
- an organizational structure that operates a division of labor (a specialization of activity) to ensure that common needs are met
- often a shared territory

Community systems are comprised of individuals, families, groups, and organizations that operate within its boundaries. However, it should be noted that not all boundaries in communities have a common physical border. Ferdinand Tonnies differentiated between "place-based communities", or physical localities, and "mind communities", in which a common identity is maintained without residing within a defined space (Anderson & Carter, 1990); examples include the LGBTQ, religious, and gaming communities. Place communities may be urban, suburban, or rural and are diverse in many other ways—mind communities may likewise have much diversity despite their shared focus. Both types may also have differing levels of organization.

Another type of community group consists of "social networks" or people who are linked together in a variety of ways—a person will normally have many of these linkages at any one time and numerous ones over a lifetime. With the advent of the internet, these connections are expanding as nonplace or mind communities are forcing systems to adapt and change in a variety of ways.

Neighborhoods are geographic areas (place communities) that exist in cities and towns and possess distinct physical boundaries that have the formal nature of official boundaries, such as deeds, tracts, and zip codes

(Hill & Maimon, 2013). For purposes of our systemic analysis, both communities and neighborhoods are systems that seek stability and that must adapt to changing conditions. As face-to-face contact is increasingly being replaced by electronic communication and online social networking, changes are occurring with mental health, at both the individual and societal levels.

As noted in chapter two, it has historically fallen to communities and neighborhoods to deal with those in their midst who exhibit mental disorders to decide what to do to assist them (although in many instances, community members sought to remove them completely). Decisions of what to do often falls to communities and neighborhoods as families are sometimes overwhelmed with the challenges in maintaining them at home and because their options seem limited. Also, transient often people drift into communities, leaving their hosts to decide actions to be taken on their behalf. Fortunately, there are service providers of different sorts in many areas, in fact, most programs for the mentally ill are outpatient community programs. Unfortunately, there are communities who lack these services, forcing people to receive them in other towns and communities (some far away), creating yet another barrier to mental health treatment.

Service delivery systems

The service delivery systems exist to assist people with a variant of needs. Providers might be private or public and could exist on different geopolitical levels—community, state, or federal. Systems in this group include the educational system, family assistance and child welfare programs, the criminal justice system, and the physical health care system. These systems are important component parts that work in tandem with the mental health system.

The educational system's primary function is, of course, the education and skills training of people at different stages of the life course to improve occupational chances and to expand people's understanding of the world. However, there are many students that would not be able to be as effective in achieving their goals without schools attending to their mental health needs. School counselors, in addition to their guidance counseling duties, frequently encounter students with emotional and substance abuse problems and must be able to confront these issues and refer when necessary. In addition, there are school-based therapists in many educational institutions that can provide services to students with greater psychological needs (Carlson & Kees, 2013).

Family assistance and child welfare systems function to ensure the safety of children through activity that promotes safe, stable home environments (Shireman, 2015). Because of the importance of family stability in the lives of children, the issue of well-being is currently a focus of child welfare programs. Programs that ensure children's mental health is important to their ability to become happy, well-functioning adults, therefore, there is a close connection to the mental health system, as well as the justice system, school systems, disability services, domestic violence programs, foster care providers, and childhood education programs.

The criminal justice system is another system that is closely connected to the mental health system. This system is comprised of three major components—the police, the courts, and corrections. Rates of arrest of the mentally ill are higher than most other groups and encounters and can be especially troublesome in terms of the stress, anxiety, and stigma produced in these encounters (Sugie & Turney, 2017).

As noted earlier, the court system often adjudicates people who have mental health and addiction problems to the extent that America now has mental health and drug courts to specifically handle people with these problems. The correctional system is the final sector of the criminal justice system (although the "revolving door" process often keeps people circulating through the system) and unfortunately people who have mental health and addiction problems end up in our nation's jails and prisons; while these have some treatment programming, they are limited and often fall short of being effective. Prisons have become "de facto mental health centers" (Brandt, 2012, p. 554), therefore adequate funding of treatment programs in prisons and jails should be of paramount importance. On a similar note, substance abuse and addiction are also on the rise and a focus on addiction treatment programs is recommended (National Center on Addiction and Substance Abuse at Columbia University, 2010). Parole and probation services are components of the correctional system and are responsible for the supervision of offenders in the community: often these agencies provide referral services to mental health and substance abuse programs outside the correctional system.

The health care system

Prior to considering the components of this massive system, we will look at the history of the general health care system to provide a more systematic view of health care, which also includes the insurance system. A historical approach also provides some insight into the current controversies over the role of the government (as opposed to the free market) in the provision of health care.

In the American colonies there was a mixture of public and private health care service provision. Towns and counties were often given the responsibility for aiding its sick, indigent citizens in the form of almshouses. These almshouses later employed physicians and eventually became hospitals. Most people during this period, however never used hospitals and instead relied on family or friends when sick or injured. Private practice physicians began to make "house calls" but their care was often substandard.

During the nineteenth century, private (or "voluntary") hospitals and those operated by religious groups sprang up in the country. The earliest form of health insurance was provided to sailors, which was later extended to veterans of the other branches in the form of what would become the Veterans Assistance (VA) hospitals after World War I. What was termed "sickness insurance" was debated in the United States political system but when America entered the war, the discussion ended when it was revealed that the first insurance program began in Germany—not a popular country at that time (Hoffman, 2012).

The prosperity that Americans experienced in the years immediately after World War I gave rise to community hospitals, which became the lynchpin of the health care system from 1920-1950. The Great Depression caused major changes as to how health care was paid. An experiment began in Dallas, Texas in which teachers in a local school district put fifty cents into a private hospital fund that gave the teachers hospital visits totaling twenty-one days annually, heralding the beginning of employer based health insurance. This arrangement soon spread to other organizations, prompted in part by labor union collective bargaining. Community hospitals were replaced by medical centers in the 1960s until 1980; these facilities provided more advanced technology and procedures which came with a hefty price tag, causing health care costs to soar. Since older Americans often did not have insurance coverage, Medicare was created by the Federal government in the mid-1960s and was soon followed by Medicaid to ensure health care coverage for low income people (Hoffman, 2012).

Health care costs rose dramatically in the 1970s and a new plan, labeled "managed care" was instituted whose purpose was to control these costs. Managed care, as represented in health management organizations (HMOs), were able to cut health care costs but the procedures used to accomplish this end limited the number of visits, dictated who would provide care, and basically placed many restrictions on both patients and medical care providers. Increased media attention spelled the end of managed care. Earlier efforts by U.S. Presidents Richard Nixon, Jimmy Carter, and Bill Clinton to move health care under national administration had failed but in 2010, President Barack Obama initiated the Patient Protection and Affordable Care Act (known primarily as the Affordable Care Act or informally as Obamacare) which moved some health care control to the government (Hoffman, 2012). The election of Donald Trump in 2016 signaled a series of steps to dismantle the Affordable Care Act. Health care, possibly more than any other social concern, represents the ideological differences in the two major political parties.

The current health system in the United States is a byzantine system and has within it five components. For example, there are medical facilities that include both inpatient and outpatient programs. There is also the workforce consisting of large number of employees who attend to those in need of medical services. The providers of therapeutics, including pharmacology and medical equipment, are another important part of the system. Educational and research centers provide empirical data to the greater health care system. And there is also the financial system that consists of the payment of medical care services. In addition to these components, there is an administrative structure that makes sure the system functions correctly (Jonas, Goldsteen, & Goldsteen, 2013).

There are many subsystems within these systems (which could themselves be considered subsystems), for example, hospitals come in different types with different systems, foci, and requirements, based on their functionality: general, special, rehabilitation/chronic, and psychiatric, all run by a variety of administrative systems at local, district, state, federal, and private levels. The different financial types include not-for-profit and private/for-profit (Jonas, Goldsteen, & Goldsteen, 2013). In addition, nursing homes, although considered in a separate category, provide residential health services. And, of course, substance abuse hospitals also administer inpatient health care as well.

These are but a few of the many systems that act interdependently within the mental health system. Others include systems that provide food assistance, housing services, employment assistance, disability services, domestic violence intervention, teen pregnancy programs, among many more— indicating the web of services that are provided through these systems are indeed colossal.

The cultural system

It is well beyond the scope and focus of this section to define the "American culture" as it comprises a huge system of national beliefs, norms values, preferences, etc., but the idea of a culture specific to America has been an appealing one for a very long time. Culture refers to the "socially shared systems of beliefs, values, and meanings" of a society (Horowitz,

2010, p. 7). These shared features of a culture require the creation of social institutions that function to deal with various needs of the society.

Many scholars have attempted to describe this esoteric idea of American culture beginning in the late 1700s, but it was Alexis de Tocqueville's *Democracy in America* (1835 & 1840/2000) that provided the first comprehensive analysis of the American dualism between individual and society (Bellah, Madsen, Sullivan, Swidler, & Tipton, 1985). The democratic spirit allowed the American citizen to participate in social institutions such as government, family, and religion while maintaining a degree of independence and individuality.

Bellah et al. (1985), in describing American culture's more rationalizing and efficiency-seeking elements, explain how the psychotherapist represents the national character through seeking a cure for the problems that afflict Americans at both micro and macro levels; the term therapeutic suggests a need for a cure—the cure being liberation and commitment that come from an individual's integration into society. Some aspects can be derived from the general American culture such as:

- individualism
- a belief in democracy
- the preference for a free market economic system
- and a belief in the benefits of technological advancement

The theme of the individual is reflected in *Habits of the Heart* (Bellah et al., 1985), which took its title from de Tocqueville's description of American mores, or deeply held traditions. It is perhaps the individualistic tradition that promotes stigma to those with mental illness; while physical illness is perceived as the result of an external event or condition, mental illness is perceived as a character flaw or an indication of a person being unable to adequately deal with the vicissitudes of life.

The underlying belief system in democratic political systems is that every citizen (within certain parameters) has a voice in constructing social conditions. Incorporated in that idea is the related concept of equality—that citizens should be treated fairly and in an equitable manner, as circumstances dictate. Although, as we have seen in our historical review in chapter two, people with mental disorders were often not treated with the respect and dignity extended to other citizens. Although this condition still exists, there has been some progress in the humane treatment of the mentally ill, and people with disabilities generally. Anchored to the democratic ideal, this progression will hopefully lead to novel strategies for advocacy as will be covered in chapter seven.

The preference for a free market system is obvious in attempts to finance mental health care. New Deal policies and the American Care Act notwithstanding, health care in America has been the purview of the free market rather than the government, unlike many other nations in the industrialized world. This reflects the American reliance on market approaches over what some consider "socialized medicine". Despite continuing problems in financing health care, including mental health care, the country is still grappling with this issue. And health care costs are still very high, and many Americas have insufficient care.

The national belief in the saving graces of technology to solve the world's problems (despite the fear of it mentioned earlier) is quite clear. For example, advances in technology that focus on brain science and other biological-related disciplines are considered by many to someday reveal the answers to adequately understand and treat mental illness (noting, of course, that these do not adequately address mental health conditions that have environmental causes). And, obviously, the advancements in psychopharmacology have led many to believe in the progress of mental health treatment based on advancements in drug creation. It could be claimed the overreliance on drug therapy, promoted by an industry obsessed with greater profits, reinforce the culture's belief in drugs to solve social problems.

An interesting idea that connects aspects of culture to mental illness can be found in the idea of symptom pools. Essentially this refers to conditions when new symptoms emerge which have an unexplained physiological origin, especially related to cultural anxiety. As Shorter (1992) notes "the surrounding culture provides our unconscious minds with templates or models of illness" (p. 2). Thus, conditions such as fits, hysteria, neurasthenia, and more recently, anorexia nervosa, as well as their treatment, are shaped by cultural explanations. The symptoms are not created by society; they are retrieved from the symptom pools that are derived from cultural understandings of the world.

The "culture-bound syndromes" that have recently been added to the DSM reflect cultural interpretations experienced by people in different parts of the world. Unexplained conditions not supported by medical knowledge use the surrounding culture to provide ideas on curious and ambiguous disorders (see Littlewood, 2002). Regarding the symptom pool thesis, this approach is based more on social constructionism than biological determinism, despite the latter's growing popularity.

The cultural system creates customs that shape the availability, quality, quantity, and type of mental services rendered to its citizens (Horowitz, 2010). The provision of these services constitutes "cultures of care" or "cultures of healing" that directly reflect the shared understandings and prescribed action of the greater culture (Fancher, 1995).

Now that we have had a comprehensive look at systems theory, it is time for a brief examination of the current mental health system in America specifically.

THE AMERICAN SYSTEM OF MENTAL HEALTH

The mental health system is comprised of consumers and those who are tasked with helping them. Consumers are engaged in both informal and formal sectors; the informal sector is comprised of the networks of nonprofessional helpers such as family, friends, self-help groups, and others, while the formal sector consists of trained mental health practitioners, such as those mentioned in chapter three. Professional mental health service provisions are delivered in both inpatient and outpatient settings.

Most therapy is provided in outpatient venues which provide services based on such factors as diagnosis, severity of presenting symptoms, to some extent, choice of provider. Outpatient services delivered in clinics involve case management services (which provide linkages to appropriate services to aid in treatment), planning for transitions through the process (including the transition from child and adolescent services to adult programming) and referrals to internal and external programs, such as AA (Polgar, 2010). The outpatient sector of the mental health system has many programs such as individual and group counseling, day treatment, other specialty programs, and of course, medication programs. Payment for services is made through private insurance or funding through government sources such as social security insurance, social security, and Medicare.

It has long been the mental hospital that represents the iconic symbol of the mental health system. A history of the asylum has been explained earlier in this book, can be found in numerous other sources, and needs little elaboration here. In contrast to its asylum predecessor, modern hospitals, despite their lower numbers, provide many programs to different groups such as rehabilitation programs, family services, various workshops, and case management (Scheid & Brown, 2010).

There is a series of core functions for mental health services that provide a useful framework for the provision of mental health services:

- initiation—the agency identifies a need and develops a strategic plan to address the need

- facilitation—the organization acts by identifying and bringing together partners to address the issue and to provide support, including financial
- dissemination—the agency provides the information and data about services, programs, and actions and develops, improves, and updates technology regarding existing methods of communication
- measurement—the center gets assessment and evaluation data on existing programs and analyzes this data for improved service provision of goal reassessment (Power, 2009).

CONCLUSION

A systems approach is beneficial in examining the mental health system as it effectively represents the interconnectivity and interrelatedness of the organizations related to mental health with those other structures that seek to make it functional. By understanding the structure and function of systems and subsystems, the role of boundaries, the flow of energy through the various systems, the activity of feedback loops, the process of individuation, and other basic features of a systems approach, we can better understand how to use this knowledge to create a better system as well as a better relationship between the systems involved with mental health care.

Systems perspectives have influenced social thinkers for eons. In nineteenth century Western society, Herbert Spencer articulated how a systems construction called organicism metaphorically allows us to see the mental health system as analogous to a machine or the human body with interrelated parts that must function appropriately for the system to remain functional or "healthy". The systems approach relates to the sociological imagination in that it sees systems at different levels—from the personal to the cultural, and it observes the interplay that exists between them.

Using general systems theory as a prototype, several models were created to illustrate the various systems that exist in our lives. The basic model adopted in this chapter examined how the mental health system can be viewed from the levels of the personal system, families and small groups, communities, service delivery systems, and the overarching cultural system.

In the mental health field, a holistic approach has been adopted. The recent focus on the integration of Eastern philosophy and spirituality, especially mindfulness, into Western treatment protocols is an example of how the interconnectivity of different perspectives can be used to promote a better functioning mental health system by using approaches of those from other cultural systems.

The premise of the social systems concept is that there is a natural organization of functions within groupings. The system of mental health, like other systems, is deemed healthy or unhealthy, just as individuals are given the same classification. The idea that systems in society resemble systems in nature provides some information about the cultural need to relate things social to things natural. This idea of a social system creates both an association between humans with nature and, at the same time, creates a distinction between them. Systems provide the idea that there is an order to society, as there is in nature. Evolutionary processes can be found in both, though at times social theory has engaged ideas of Social Darwinism that classifies and socially stratifies people. Fortunately, current understandings of differences in race, ethnicity, gender, identity, and other classifications have evidenced a substructure that values the "treatment" of people on equitable grounds. That this value has not been adopted more fully in our society is troubling, but an understanding of our history tells us this social evolution towards equality is continuing, albeit slowly.

Chapter 7

STRATEGIES FOR MENTAL HEALTH ADVOCACY

> "...madness is the false punishment of a false solution, but by its own virtue, it brings to light the real problems, which can then be truly resolved"
>
> (Michel Foucault, 1988 p. 33)

ADVOCACY DEFINED

Advocacy in the mental health field has a long history. The word itself has its roots in fourteenth century Europe and originally referred to legal representation. There were several key people and key legislative actions since that time to assist people in dealing with the mental health system in an advocacy role. Advocacy in mental health is rapidly growing not only in the United States but also Australia, Canada, Europe, New Zealand, and many other countries (World Health Organization, 2003).

A definition of advocacy is "the process of identifying with and representing a person's views and concerns, in order to secure enhanced rights and entitlements, undertaken by someone who has little or no conflict of interest" (Henderson & Pochin, 2001, p. 1-2). It is "the act of pleading or arguing in favor of something, such as a cause, idea, or policy. It is about opening doors and making friends to get your message across" (Ptakowski, 2012, p.51). In mental health advocacy, supporters must clearly identify the problem, research the problem fully, then proceed to argue their case. Some strategies in this regard will be addressed soon.

According to the World Health Organization (WHO), an important resource in providing awareness to governments of the world on the concerns of mental illness, advocacy can result in better policy, legislation and service outcomes in mental health care. In addition, it can lead to a reduction in stigma and discrimination against people deemed mentally ill. In recent years advocacy has evolved to include the needs of people with less severe mental conditions and for the needs of those in the general population. Advocacy activity includes:

- the promotion of awareness
- information dissemination
- education and training
- counseling and mutual help
- mediating, supporting, and denouncing (WHO, 2003)

Advocacy is not of one type—there are many types that exist to assist people in creating better life conditions:

- collective advocacy, which refers to people championing a cause either individually or as a group
- community advocacy, a special type of collective advocacy, which is often used if the cause affects a specific group
- professional advocacy, in which people who are employed in a professional capacity speak up for those for whom they provide services
- peer advocacy, a type in which people with similar circumstances support a cause
- legal advocacy, which, as the name implies, connotes the provision of legal representation on causes of concern
- citizen advocacy, a long term, unpaid collaboration on a vulnerable person's behalf
- non-instructed advocacy, which occurs when someone advocates for people who are unable to speak for themselves
- self-advocacy, in which people with a cause speak for themselves to promote change (Newbigging et al., 2015)

There is obviously some overlap between these types; for example, one can see how a citizen advocate could also be functioning as a non-instructed advocate if their "partner" (a term for the person for whom the advocacy is being sought), is incapacitated or otherwise unable to advocate for themselves.

Advocates of mental health include a wide variety of specific groups including consumers and their families, health practitioners, politicians, and civil libertarians, ensuring that advocacy is often driven by competing agendas and sometimes irreconcilable differences (WHO, 2003).

The World Health Organization (WHO) is actively engaged with countries to "place mental health on the public agenda, to promote a greater acceptance of persons with mental disorders, to protect their human rights, and to reduce the pervasive effects of stigma" (2003, p.15). They have been successful in applying pressure to countries to improve services for the mentally ill (Kelly, 2009). WHO has aided the mentally ill, their families, and professional agencies and organizations and has taken an active role in engaging the public in mental health advocacy. However, the agency recognizes certain barriers:

- poor quality of care or lack of appropriate services
- the high cost of mental health care
- lack of parity with physical health care
- too few consumer-run services
- lack of a collaborative effort between consumers and providers
- human rights violations
- inadequate housing
- stigma
- lack of advocacy and prevention services in schools, workplaces, and communities
- lack of sufficient mental health programs globally (WHO, 2003)

Despite the barriers, the benefits of advocacy are well worth the work it takes to break these barriers. Even though there exists no definitive data about benefits, positive outcomes that result from advocacy include:

- greater visibility of mental health concerns at the governmental level
- improvement of mental health treatment, prevention policies, and practices
- positive change regarding laws and governmental policies
- protection and promotion of the rights of the mentally ill
- improvement of services (WHO, 2003)

A SHORT HISTORY OF MENTAL HEALTH ADVOCACY

Different people, events, and organizations in the cyclic model that was discussed in chapter two had different levels of advocacy, or what passed for advocacy. Advocacy activity initially involved communities working together to assist the vulnerable citizens in their communities and to combat the stigma experienced by the mad among them (WHO, 2003).

Several groups have been suggested as the first mental health advocacy organization. One involved a group of people who in the seventeenth century protested the treatment of patients in the infamous Bedlam. Other candidates included physicians from the eighteenth century and early nineteenth century who advocated for mental patients. Or perhaps the award belongs to eighteenth-century Scotch publisher Alexander Cruden who advocated mental health reform (Newbigging et al., 2015). Another possibility was a group called the Alleged Lunatics' Friends Society (ALFS), who in the nineteenth century pressured policy makers to create reforms for the mentally ill (Burns, 2006; Newbigging et al., 2015).

As we saw in earlier chapters, what is termed the era of moral treatment began in 1795 with several "madhouse managers", including British Quaker William Tuke, French physician Phillipe Pinel, as well as other proponents of this new idea of better treatment of mental health inmates through humane conduct. Tuke founded the Retreat in York that had a physical environment meant to rectify some of the harsh conditions encountered by the mentally ill during this time by creating an environment that consisted of a humane environment with good rapport between staff (including administration) and patients—this model was later recreated in America. Phillipe Pinel, a former medical writer who experienced the death of a mentally ill friend, used his grief to move into the asylum system and create changes (Lieberman, 2015). In the tenuous zeitgeist of post-Revolutionary Paris, Pinel systematically made changes to two major hospitals. Like Tuke in England, he believed the institution was the best place to create positive change, away from the deleterious influences of family and acquaintances outside the hospital, by providing an atmosphere of acceptance and encouragement (Scull, 2015). While there were many key players in the moral treatment phase, they all had commonalities: the asylum administration by one key, benevolent parent-like figure; rewards for work and self-control; trust and reciprocal behavior between administration and inmate; and generally, a warm environment akin to what is referred to as "supportive" in the mental health field today (Johnson, 1990).

Thomas Story Kirkbride is also credited with developing the moral reform movement in America. Like Tuke, Kirkbride was a Quaker who sought to improve the lives of asylum inmates at mid-nineteenth century. His book *On the Construction, Organization, and General Arrangement of Hospitals for the Insane*, published in 1854, became the standard guide for the construction and operation of mental institutions. He stressed routine, order, and supervision though his prisons took on the appearance of incarceration facilities. Kirkbride believed the mad were curable and deserving of appropriate therapeutic methods that set the standard of care in the era (Mintz, 1995).

Benjamin Rush, mentioned many times already, was a true advocate for the mentally ill and substance abusers. He believed that insanity had increased at the end of the 1700s due to a social obsession with money and the consequences of the new banking system (Torrey & Miller, 2001). He also imported the moral treatment movement from Europe to the United States (Johnson, 1990). Although Rush continued to use the "modern" therapeutics learned from his European teachers such as bleeding, spinning, numerous methods to re-direct blood from an over-heated brain and through the use of his own creation, the infamous tranquilizer chair, he also brought the European hospital model to Philadelphia where he was physician and faculty member. His advocacy for mental health patients, despite his unorthodox treatments, eventually resulted in improved conditions for American mental patients (Whitaker, 2002). And although Rush was a moral reformer, he is primarily remembered for his work on temperance. While alcohol had been regarded as a moral force by many early Americans, Rush wrote several tracts on the benefits of remaining alcohol free and produced a "moral and physical thermometer" that illustrated his ideas on the social, medical, and moral consequences of alcoholism. Rush's advocacy was, of course, for abstinence and prevention, with the hope of producing a more moral and functional America that would emerge when addiction would be viewed as a disease capable of being cured (Lender & Martin, 1987).

Dorothea Dix is one of the most well-known of all mental health advocates and activists. Having survived major depressive symptoms as a young woman, she was sent to live with a family in England who were descendants of reformer William Tuke. Trained in the Quaker framework and moral treatment model, she returned home and furiously advocated for institutions of the European type to be instituted in the United States. Appealing to politicians, she was able to gather support for the idea of humane asylums that removed the mentally ill from institutions that also housed criminals (Whitaker, 2002). She teamed up with political reformer Horace Mann in the mid-1800s to create the Dix-Mann formula for hospital care programs, with funding from the federal level to be transferred to the states. Dix successfully persuaded politicians in all states to adopt her asylum model. After getting politicians from all the United States onboard, she went to Scotland to promote her ideas on "lunacy reform" (Scull, 2015, p.196).

The mental hygiene movement provided a major push for mental health advocacy. While this movement had several key people, Clifford Beers was one of its most vocal representatives. Beers was drawn to advocacy due to his own mental condition, probably bipolar disorder, as well as the poor treatment he received as a hospital patient. He was able to attract attention to mental hygiene to big names such as psychologist/philosopher William James, who provided financial support, and renowned psychiatrist Adolf Meyer, who assisted with his writing. When asked by Meyer to tone down his anti-psychiatry rhetoric, Beers refused and the two parted ways. In his famous autobiographical work, *A Mind that Found Itself* (1935), he stated the work was not meant as entertainment but rather "the opening gun in a permanent campaign for improvement" (Beers, 1935, p.255), a campaign that sought to improve mental health problems and to prevent them when possible. Beers became a salesman for mental hygiene and successfully created a national movement, propelled by an organization called the National Committee for Mental Hygiene, for which Beers became its secretary and primary advocate (Porter, 2002). He continued to work within the movement until he was returned to institutional life in 1939, dying in a mental hospital a few years later (Johnson, 1990).

In the field of substance abuse advocacy, few people have had the influence of AA founders Bill W and Dr. Bob, mentioned earlier in this book. Through their work, they reached out to many people, published a guide for sobriety (the Big Book) with steps and traditions, and worked out a strategy that soon became a movement—the twelve-step program of AA. Their reach extended outside of the United States and to the world and is one of the world's largest advocacy groups.

Another interesting chapter in the field of mental health advocacy involves the work of conscientious objectors (COs) who during World War II were opposed to military service on moral or religious grounds. The COs were allowed to work in hospitals during the war in lieu of fighting in combat. These individuals, who were often highly educated and morally upright, were appalled at the conditions witnessed in the mental hospitals. An organization was formed by a group of COs called the National Mental Health Foundation (NMHF) to establish an advocacy program that was similar to the mental hygiene programs. Riding the post-war wave for social betterment, several advocacy organizations were formed, including the National Institute for Mental Health (NIMH), which was created by consolidating existing programs including Beers' National Commission for Mental Hygiene, the American Psychological Foundation, as well as the conscientious objectors' NMHF. The NIMH obtained prominence as an advocacy group beginning in the 1950s and continuing to today (Johnson, 1990).

During the post-World War II period, there was another push for changes in the mental health system. As Johnson (1990) puts it, "the public's conscience about its mentally ill underwent one of its periodic shakeups" (p. 25). This time, news accounts of asylum life shook the national conscience as journalist Albert Deutsch published his findings, including graphic images, about the deleterious conditions of the era's prisons. Deutsch, who had earlier published a book called *The Mentally Ill in America* (1935) that was often used as a source of historical information, published another work called *The Shame of the States* (1948) that was extremely beneficial in calling attention to the problems in the nation's institutions (Johnson, 1990; Scull, 2015). Deutsch made comparisons of American asylums to the Nazi death camps and these were obviously made in response to the eugenics movement that had become a part of the national mental health landscape as well (Whitaker, 2015). It should be noted that other forms of media also informed the public of the toxic conditions of the hospitals; popular novels such as 1946's *The Snake Pit*, 1962's *One Flew Over the Cuckoo's Nest*, and 1963's *The Bell Jar*, and later movie versions of the same names, exposed this information to a large audience of readers and viewers (Scull 2015).

Less well known than Tuke, Pinel, Kirkbride, Beers, Deutsch, and certainly Rush and Dix, Barbara Robb was an English psychotherapist who contributed substantially to advocacy and deserves mention. Robb, who was investigating an asylum near London became upset at the conditions she observed and kept a diary of her experiences, describing patient maltreatment and the lack of concern, activities, and respect from the understaffed institution. She formed a pressure group to force the British government to make changes in the system; this group went by the name Aid for the Elderly in Governmental Institutions (AEGIS). Robb wrote a book called *Sans Everything: A Case to Answer* which was published by AEGIS and detailed her accounts of patient abuse and neglect. Robb's expose did not sit well with the British government and the backlash was extreme. She would later be vindicated and her whistle blowing activity created a counterweight to the inhumane practices in psychiatric hospitals (Hilton, 2017)

Betty Ford was an unlikely advocate for substance addiction and other mental disorders. First Lady and wife of Gerald Ford, the 38th President of the United States, she was an advocate for many causes, including women's equality and substance abuse treatment. She was also addicted to alcohol and prescription medications. She went into recovery and in 1982 founded the Betty Ford Clinic (now Center), which became a nationally acclaimed addiction program. The fact than many celebrities have attended the clinic made the issue of addiction less secretive.

It depends on one's point of view to determine if the group described as the anti-psychiatrists would be considered as advocates for the mentally ill. They did speak out on behalf of this group in response to what they thought was a system that was unfair to them. As mentioned in chapter two, Thomas Szasz, R.D. Laing, Irving Goffman, and Thomas Sheff all approached this advocacy in different ways, but all felt the state of psychiatry at the time was harming the mentally ill. Currently, a similar stance has been taken by a group of practitioners and scholars that feel the DSM and psychopharmacology are the enemies of good mental health practice.

Rosalynn Carter became involved in mental health issues when her husband, Jimmy Carter, became a Georgia gubernatorial candidate (he would, of course, later became the 39th President of the United States). Ms. Carter was asked about her candidate husband's plans for addressing the needs of the mentally ill and afterward educated herself on the subject by observing facilities and talking with staff and consumers. When President Carter took office, Rosalynn became secretary of the newly formed President's Commission on Mental Health. The problems brought about by deinstitutionalization, the communities' lack of preparation to deal with it, and inadequate mental health financing, were to be addressed and research, prevention, and disability services were planned. These plans were scrapped when the next presidential administration entered the White House. The Carter Center was founded in Georgia in the 1980s with the aim of addressing a variety of social problems and continues to seek reforms that benefit the mentally ill and actively reduce the stigma of mental illness (Carter, 1999).

There are many different people who could have been added to this section of advocates. The ones chosen in the previous section represent a wide variety of people—alienists, activists, asylum managers, physicians, writers, people with political ties, mental health consumers, and various other groups. They represent the different types of advocacy mentioned in the introductory paragraph of this chapter. And they all sought, in different ways, to make things better for those with mental disorders. And hopefully, they will serve as examples we can emulate to create change in our own time.

MULTICULTURALISM AND SOCIAL JUSTICE IN ADVOCACY

Multiculturalism is mentioned in this section as mental illness is not a problem with any certain segment of society, but all segments. Multicultural counseling can be defined as therapeutic work with clients with an understanding of the cultural differences that exist between different people. A similar term, cultural competence, is used to describe this culturally relative approach to understanding differences. George Herbert Mead's concept of taking the role of the other is relevant here as practitioners are expected to not only be aware of differences but to have a subjective understanding of how clients are experiencing mental distress. It is only through attempts to understand the concerns of mental health consumers that mental health therapists will be able to create positive treatment outcomes.

Social justice is defined as an ideal that seeks to create equality in laws and in social institutions, including the health care system, in a manner that "is guided by the moral principles of truth, reason, justice and fairness" (Badley, 1996, p. 73). In the mental health care institution, social justice can include these goals:

- the reduction of stigma
- the provision of health care parity that is in line with physical care
- better access to accommodations and treatment services (Badley, 1996).

It is social justice that has driven the mental health advocates and activists throughout history.

In the counseling field, a focus on multiculturalism and social justice has been a major goal for the several years. Recently, a set of standards to meet this end, the Multicultural and Social Justice Counseling Competencies (MSJCC) replaced an earlier set of standards that failed to adequately emphasize the social justice component. Utilizing the concept of intersectionality—the overlapping of identities such as those involving race, gender, sexuality, socioeconomics, age, and disability, which occur in varying degrees, the MSJCC seeks to develop cultural and social justice. Noting the effects of identity not only on the patient but also on the therapist and the community is an important part of this new focus. Understanding the role of addressing oppression in advocacy for those marginalized people with mental illness reflects the social justice component of the MSJCC (Ratts, Singh, Nassar-McMillan, Butler, & McCullough, 2016).

ADVOCACY FOR SPECIAL GROUPS

In the spirit of multiculturalism and social justice, we will now look at advocacy concerns for some selected groups. These are certainly not indicative of all groups, but they provide a sampling that can be useful in considering advocacy for people with mental health needs.

Addicted persons

One way that practitioners can promote substance abuse advocacy is through what is known as program evaluation, in which addiction programs are closely examined to ensure they are meeting expected outcomes regarding treatment and prevention. The information from evaluation can then be used to advocate in areas that are considered best practices. Areas that can be considered in completing evaluation are:

- specific needs of minority populations with addiction issues
- barriers to effective assessment of treatment services
- interventions for specific addictions
- descriptive and outcome research information
- support, including funding, from involved stakeholders for the provision of services to underserved people (Astramovich & Hoskins, 2013).

A growing concern in the substance abuse field is a crisis involving people addicted to opioids. The opioid crisis is a bit different from some other drug scares in the past as this one began with the abuse of pain medication which became a national epidemic (Hodge, Wetter, & Noe, 2017). People with addictions have been labeled throughout history as “dope fiends”, “junkies”, “dope heads” “crack mothers” (among many others) and stereotyped as violent, aggressive, and antisocial; these labels and stereotypes have often created barriers for them to receive appropriate treatment. It seems people addicted to opioid pain medications have so far been exempt from some of these labels at this point and are even seen as victims in many instances; this might change, however, as time passes.

Women

Throughout history, women have been perceived as possessing major differences from men regarding mental health and health generally. Men’s bodily constitution was perceived as the norm while women possessed bodies that were “fundamentally inferior: moister, looser textured, softer, with spongier flesh” (Scull, 2009, p.13). Of special concern was the womb, which was considered by Hippocrates, and many other men of medicine, to be the origin of all disease. The womb, it was posited, was an organ that wandered around inside the female body seeking moisture. Women’s bodies naturally needed to have blood released (through bloodletting, of course) due to excessive amounts of liquid in the body (Scull, 2009). In times when witches were suspected of causing all manner of social distress, demons were believed to enter women’s bodies quite easily. And much later when poor parenting was determined to be the cause of schizophrenia and other mental disorders, it was the mother who was determined to be the reason for the problem. The fragility of the female constitution was highlighted in certain disorders, such as hysteria and neurasthenia, that seemed to be tailor-made for delicate upper-class ladies.

Since females were not taken seriously in scholarly pursuits, they often did not get their work published or have their voices heard. One of those who fought to be heard, Charlotte Perkins Gilman, was a sociologist who produced searing insights into gender relations in America at the turn of the 20th century. She is perhaps best known, however, as the author of a short story published in the nineteenth century titled *The Yellow Wallpaper* (1892) which described a woman's slow retreat into depression and psychosis, revealing the special concerns of gender as it relates to mental illness.

In 1968, as women's issues were beginning to be addressed at the dawn of the "women's liberation" movement, Chesler, in her study of female mental patients, described the "female 'career' as a psychiatric patient in America" as following "a certain pattern as a function of age, marital status, social class, race, and most certainly 'attractiveness'" (1972, p.120). Understanding gender differences is important in the mental health field because certain mental disorders are exclusively found in women, such as premenstrual dysmorphic disorder and postpartum depression, and some are more common such as anxiety, depression and eating disorders (NIMH, 2016). But while some disorders have a biological feature, females have long experienced social stressors differently than males due to gender roles expectations and the treatment of women generally; often these conditions were chalked up to the delicate and fragile (we should read: inferior) female constitution, as noted earlier. Great strides have been made in the pursuit of gender equality and other women's issues (as represented in the recent Women's March, Me, Too and Times Up movements), however, it would be extremely naïve to believe fairness has been achieved.

Children

A 2009 summit on children's mental health concerns acknowledged two related barriers to children and adolescent services—the current economic situation (which, it should be noted has improved since that time), and budget cuts on local levels (which seem to always be a problem). Some advocacy programs (Odar, Canter, & Roberts, 2013) for children are recommended that involve:

- the provision of social and emotional support
- a better understanding of the benefits of a stable home environment and set routines
- an increase in knowledge about child developmental processes
- skills training in working with children and families to produce better mental health outcomes

A recent advance in this area can be found in the Internet's potential to provide information on child and adolescent issues (Odar, Canter, & Roberts, 2013).

The "sturm and drang" of adolescence, the stormy, stressful period of teenage hormonal and social vagaries are well known, especially by parents. But beyond the "normal misery of adolescence" (Scarf, 1980, p. 21) of feeling different, odd, awkward, unaccepted, and sometimes out of control, there are young people who experience the additional stress and stigma of mental illness and addiction. Growing pains of adolescence normally pass without major incident, but for others, there are lifelong adjustments. The growing concern of school shootings also promotes greater anxiety among children and this is an area that should be addressed in more detail.

Racial and ethnic minorities

Poor mental and physical health outcomes are associated with people of racial and ethnic minority status due to a long history of systemic and structural oppression and marginalization (Bowen & Walton, 2015). People often misuse the terms race and ethnicity—race refers to biological characteristics that have been lumped together and given special significance; modern sociological understandings of race involve the idea of race as being socially constructed, however, even though it is not a distinct biological reality, racial difference is real in its consequences—this is, as we recall, the Thomas theorem (Thomas & Thomas, 1928). Ethnicity refers to the cultural aspects (such as language, religion, traditions) of one's identity that has been passed down by custom. People of racial groups and ethnic groups have been subjected to both individual and institutional prejudice and discrimination as well as stereotyping.

Related issues such as income, educational, and occupational disparities worsen the effects of racial and ethnic prejudice and discussion. Issues for these groups include prisonization for African Americans and Latin Americans, historical trauma for Native Americans, and barriers based on language and culture for Asian Americans. In addition, arrest for substances of abuse such as marijuana are higher for blacks than whites—which is primarily the result of enhanced criminal justice supervision of minority communities. Selective enforcement techniques often result in "DWB"—Driving While Black (or Brown)—and other forms of racial/ethnic profiling.

People in the LGBTQ community

LGBTQ is a category that includes people who are lesbian, gay, bisexual, transgender, or questioning (of one's sexual or gender identity). Although this is certainly not a monolithic group, LGBTQ individuals do face certain barriers to mental health care. For example, people in this category experience:

- high rates of discrimination in the form of bullying in school
- disparities in employment
- denial of medical treatment and health care benefits
- abusive treatment in incarceration facilities
- family rejection and safety problems in the home (Castrol & Fritchle, 2013).

Stigma is very prominent in this population and internalized negative self-image can lead to a host of problems including homelessness, drug addiction, and suicide. Advocacy could include the compiling of diverse individuals and groups in the community to include LGBTQ people to help regain acceptance and security. Community-based projects can have long-term mental health benefits for this "hidden minority" (Castrol & Fritchle, 2013).

Those with suicidal ideation

The importance of establishing successful suicide prevention programs is obvious. Advocacy programs that target people who contemplate taking their own lives should be a growing national initiative. The recent suicide deaths of celebrities, including television and movie personalities Robin Williams and Anthony Bourdain, have shined additional light on the problem.

Emile Durkheim, in one of sociology's first scientific studies (1951/1897), discussed how suicide, an action that would seemingly fall under the purview of psychology, can be studied sociologically. Retrieving data from a variety of different countries, Durkheim found that levels of social integration—the level of closeness to others—can be a factor in suicide. Advocacy programs that target suicide use the same idea that positive relations to others can be a protective factor in most cases.

Most of us are familiar with suicide as the immediate ending of a life, but another type of suicide has been described called subtle suicide (Church & Brooks, 2009). This refers to a long-term condition characterized by problematic and self-destructive behaviors that reduce quality, and often length, of life. People who commit this type of suicide do not experience thoughts and feelings that contribute to a clearly defined end of life, but they do behave, consciously or unconsciously, in ways that hasten the end of life before a traditional suicide can take place. These people are the "living dead" who enter a downward spiral that alienates others and disrupts the potential saving grace of positive social attachments. Actions involved with addictive processes (with alcohol and other drugs, gambling, risky sexual behavior, or overeating) are often part of this type of suicide.

One program that targets college students at risk for suicide uses a "peer-to-peer" strategy to deter suicide. The program, known as Active Minds, addresses suicide, the second leading cause of death in this population, by using the resource of a student's peers, since these are the people most likely to realize when changes in behavior might point to a propensity to kill themselves. Registered student groups encourage discussion about mental illness in the hope that stigma will be diminished on college campuses and help will be sought. While the program uses peer-to-peer relationships to achieve its goals, it is *not* a peer-to-peer counseling program or a support group, but rather a club that advocates addressing potential mental health problems and making referrals. Active Minds has many intriguing stigma reduction programs to catch the interest of students and direct them to professional help. It is estimated that in the first ten years of its existence, the program has influenced over a million students and their families (Walther, Abelson, & Malmon, 2014). You will find contact information on this group in chapter nine.

THE SPECIAL ROLE OF STIGMA

As mentioned earlier, stigma of the mentally ill was one of the reasons advocacy programs began (WHO, 2003). Stigma refers to a characteristic possessed by someone that "causes them to have a deeply compromised social standing, a mark of shame or discredit" (WHO, 2003, p. 11). Sociologist Erving Goffman (1963) described stigma as a discrediting mark or certain attribute that creates a "spoiled identity". He stated, "(the stigmatized person) is thus reduced in our minds from a whole and usual person to a tainted, disconnected one…it is also called a failing, a shortcoming, a handicap" (Goffman, 1963 p. 3). This negative view can result in the ostracism, marginalization, and other forms of maltreatment of the mentally ill.

While Americans hold a broader understanding of mental illness than in the past, stigma continues to be a dominant force as people still tend to avoid mentally ill people and contribute violence as a major part of mental illness as they did 50 years ago (Frank & Glied, 2006). Stigma has long been a concern to sociologists. The closely related issue of labeling refers to the fact that when people are assigned a certain designation, a process is set in place where labeled people are perceived by others in a certain way. Labeling can occur in two forms: unofficial and official (Link & Phelan, 2013). Unofficial labeling refers to the everyday, informal categorization of people; official labeling occurs when some established sanctioning process takes place—such as when someone receives a DSM diagnosis from a licensed therapist. Many sociologists liken the application of a label to the creation of a deviant identity.

Lemert (1967) distinguished between primary and secondary deviance: primary deviance exists when a person commits an act that has already been labeled as deviant by authorities and secondary deviance happens when an official designating process occurs and when the stigmatizing label is internally accepted. Labeling theorists like Thomas Sheff (1966) believe the internalized label and the prejudiced gaze of others drive the mentally ill behavior. Due to convincing contradictory research evidence to this claim, a modified labeling theory was introduced that posits the label might not contribute directly to mentally disordered behavior, but the label does contribute to the mentally ill's employment chances, interpersonal relationships, and their self-esteem; these indirect consequences thwart better mental health outcomes (Link & Phelan, 2013).

Stigma exists for several reasons, including:

- to distinguish between types and levels of these differences (such as "sane" and "insane")
- to associate differences that are perceived as negative (such as the stereotypical propensity for violence)
- to separate "us" from "them" (our type of people vs. "others")
- to create an emotional response (anger, pity, and others)
- to promote a loss of social status and to discriminate against
- to claim a degree of power over those without such power (Link & Phelan, 2013)

Therefore, mental health stigma is a major reason the mentally ill do not get the care they deserve. WHO offers some ways to combat the deleterious effects of stigma:

- community and family psychoeducation on mental health stigma
- provision of training for teachers and health care providers
- empowerment of advocacy organizations
- improvement of services and social integration
- pro-mental health legislation
- education to media outlets (WHO, 2003)

The issue of "othering" is one of the causes of stigma. The term refers to placing someone outside one's own social category (which comprises many different classifications such as gender, race and ethnicity, social class, sexual identity). Othering is a two-step process: first a clear distinction is made between two categories—"us and them"; then there comes an identification of the "othered" people as outside the norm and the "othering" group as normal (Singer & Page, 2014). When someone becomes an other, it becomes easier to justify ideas of prejudice and to discriminate against them. When people become othered, or marginalized, advocates are needed to assist them.

A distinction is made between public stigma and self-stigma: public stigma refers to the stigmatized view of a group of people based on stereotypes and prejudice whereas self-stigma reflects the negative views a group of people has of themselves by accepting those negative views of others (Corrigan & Kleinlein, 2005). When there is a co-occurrence of mental illness and substance use disorder, stigmatization is amplified at both levels. And since there tends to exist differing models of treatment orientation for mental illness and addiction, there often results in a struggle over the appropriate treatment strategy (Rasinski, Woll, & Cooke, 2005). The author of this book has observed personally the conflicts between mental health and substance use treatment providers as a common occurrence.

Another type of stigma is known as structural stigma, which has generated a rapidly growing field of interest in public health (Pugh, Hatzenbuehler, & Link, 2015). Structural stigma refers to the "societal level conditions, cultural norms, and institutional practices that constrain the opportunities, resources, and wellbeing for stigmatized populations" (Hatzenbuehler & Link, 2015, p. 2). In other words, there are cultural and institutional barriers that keep the mentally ill from being able to experience the rights and benefits most people enjoy. For example, service providers sometimes promote obstacles to healthcare (especially in the form of parity in insurance coverage), education opportunities, occupational prospects, and many others. Segregation in housing areas separated from others and rejection from community members for allowing mental health facilities outright (called NIMBY for Not In My Back Yard) are other examples. As has been noted, the criminal justice system is ill-equipped to appropriately deal with the mentally ill (Pugh, Hatzenbuehler, & Link, 2015). Structural stigma may be intentional, in which people and institutions purposefully impose barriers to service provision, or unintentional in which these impositions are not intended but detrimental just the same (Livingston, 2013).

When people with mental illness are perceived as "unhealthy", biases and discrimination can occur, even if unintended, therefore poor health itself is stigmatizing and can lead to policy-making based on dislike and disdain rather than reasoned deliberation and scientific data (Roberts & Weeks, 2007). Institutional mental health discrimination is similar in many ways to institutionalized racism, sexism, or classism, and is closely associated with these characteristics, especially if the mental health stigma is compounded with other factors.

Institutional stigma of mental health can take many forms. In addition to the NIMBY factor, when mental illness is stigmatized, less money is awarded to fund research in this area. In addition, the fact that money and prestige normally go to therapists in private practice who treat the less severe clients (the "worried well"), those with more severe mental problems often are subjected to the insults of institutional stigma (Link & Phelan, 2001). There is a wealth of research data on the concept of stigma, including not only the types we have discussed, but also findings that explain how mental health stigma is experienced, perceived, internalized, and anticipated (see Fox et al., 2017).

There is an additional stigmatic element with substance use disorders because of the "war on drugs"—the idea that those addicted to substances and behaviors "brought this on themselves" and thus own the responsibility for their deviant state. Recently, the opioid epidemic which gained national attention presents a more complicated picture in that many of the opioids which caused addiction and record numbers of overdose were prescribed by physicians for other serious medical conditions. This has created two classifications—the "deserving patients" and "undeserving patients", the latter bearing the heavier burden of stigma (Buchman, Leece & Orkin, 2017).

It has been suggested we should examine the language in the mental health system. For example, the implications in the term currently in increased use "opioid overdose crisis" seems to focus on the problems of errors in dosage rather than the ingestion of the drug and the physical consequences of that ingestion; perhaps the term "opioid poisoning" is preferable to reflect the degree of responsibility and control of the person experiencing it, as opposed to other health-related issues (Buchman, Leece, & Orkin, 2017).

THE CRIMINALIZATION OF MENTAL ILLNESS

A major issue that certainly needs advocacy involves the criminalization of the mentally ill. The criminalization of mental illness refers to a social process that defines mental illness as an act of deviance to addressed by the criminal justice system rather than a psychiatric definition unique to that person (Erickson & Erickson, 2008).

It was mentioned earlier that jails and prisons have become de facto mental health institutions and this is a problem that needs to be addressed. The movement of patients from the asylums to the community ended up in the transfer of people to the streets and then to jails and prisons, a process that has been referred to as "transcarceration" (Torrey, 1997). As a result, a revolving door phenomenon has occurred which keeps the mentally ill between the streets and incarceration facilities.

The criminalization of mental illness has many consequences for society, including acts of victimization that could have been prevented by a greater focus on three issues:

- health
- the inhumane treatment of people based on them being perceived as criminal
- the lack of training of people who work in corrections that could result in assisting the mentally ill (Erickson & Erickson 2008)

Mentally ill criminal offenders can be of five different types (Hiday & Burns, 2010):

- those who commit minor, nuisance offenses including those such as disturbing the peace or loitering
- those who commit "survival behaviors" such as stealing food or other necessities
- the mentally ill who have comorbid substance use disorders and who, in addition to using illegal substances, engage in other illegal behaviors related to alcohol and other drug use such as stealing or using prostitution to obtain the substances
- those who have severe mental illness, primarily the personality disorders, and who have high rates of violent activity and substance use; this group, who often obtain the unofficial label "soci-

opath" can be aggressive and often fail to receive appropriate services due to their behavior

- the small group of mentally ill offenders that are psychotic and commit deviant or delinquent acts due to hallucinations and delusions; this group, the stereotypical "madman or madwoman" receives much media attention despite its small size

CONCLUSION

Advocacy refers to identifying with and representing a person, cause, or idea and pleading or arguing in favor of them. The World Health Organization (WHO) states there are many barriers to creating a strong system of advocacy for mental health, however, there are many positive benefits of this advocacy and it is certainly a worthwhile endeavor to be a voice for people who are often unable, or at least lack enough political power, to speak up for themselves.

There has been a long history of advocacy for people with mental illness. Practitioners, mental health consumers, activists, writers, political figures, and various other people and groups (some well-known in the field and others that are unfamiliar) have all made key contributions in the field of advocacy, from different perspectives and with different advocacy strategies. The common concern of these disparate groups has been with the welfare of people with mental illness.

Multiculturalism and social justice are major components in advocating for the mentally ill. A multicultural, or culturally competent focus in counseling, means working with clients while understanding cultural differences, their situations, and their emotional states from their perspective. Social justice is an ideal that seeks to create equality in laws and in social institutions, including the mental health care system. In mental health, the reduction of stigma, the provision of health care parity that is in line with physical care, and the access to better accommodations and treatment services have all been goals of advocacy.

There are several groups that deserve some special consideration in advocacy activity. Of these, people with addictions, women, children, racial and ethnic minorities, people in the LGBTQ community, and those with suicidal ideation all have specific treatment needs. As with multicultural counseling, an understanding and subjective appraisal of people of different types is needed by practitioners in the mental health field.

One of the greatest barriers to the welfare of those with mental problems is stigma. Stigma refers to a mark that clearly identifies someone as having unacceptable traits and who should be ostracized, marginalized, and othered. This stigmatization creates conditions for prejudice and discrimination, often requiring the assistance of advocates to promote social justice.

A pressing problem in the mental health system is the criminalization of the mentally ill. This happens when mental illness is defined by society as deviance rather than a condition needing treatment. Portrayals of the mentally ill as sociopathic killers only adds to the stigma of this population.

Even though treatment of the mentally ill throughout the world's history did not always result in favorable outcomes (or, in many cases, produced bad or very bad ones), societies have continued to support those who experience mental illness. Advocacy proves that a significant portion of our therapeutic substructure involves altruism; time, effort, expense, and other sacrifices, often great, have been made to protect the mentally ill by common citizens or those who desire to work with mental illness as an occupation. The desire to ensure that healing and fair treatment is provided to those who often have a difficult time advocating for themselves reflects some of the better features of our culture.

Chapter 8

CONCLUDING THOUGHTS

"...mental health care is fundamentally part of the public conversation that constitutes life in our society, and its recommendations are essentially moral and social programs."

(Fancher 1995, p. 5).

WHERE WE ARE: THE CRISIS OF OUR OWN AGE

The problem of mental illness in present day America is a major one—as mentioned in the introductory chapter, over 43 million Americans (about 18% of all aged 18 or over) are experiencing some degree of mental impairment and almost 10 million people (4%) of this age group are experiencing disorders that are considered severe. Mental illness among young people is certainly a concern: in the 13- to 18-year age group, over 46% have some type of mental disorder and 21% have a severe condition. Over 8 million people have co-occurring mental health and substance use disorders (NIMH, n.d.). These numbers tell us that we are all affected by mental disorders in some way, either through personal experience or with others that we know. And we have all experienced problems in living that have caused emotional distress and a decline in psychological and social functioning.

Mental health becomes an issue in mass society when some event or social condition brings it out in the open. Often acts of violence, frequently horrendous, jolt average Americans into a mindset where attention, often long overdue, is paid. As Americans are continually exposed to news events in which "mental health" is viewed as the culprit (such as mass murder or suicide), legislators and political pundits are quick to advocate increased mental health services. But funding never comes.

Frequently people with mental health problems are inappropriately portrayed as violent, out of control criminals. While it is more common for people with psychosis, especially when co-occurring with substance addictions, to commit violence than the general population, most mentally ill people do not engage in acts of violence; in fact, the mentally ill are eleven times more likely to be violently victimized than the general population (Insel, 2011). The issue of mental illness normally appears in the news after an incidence of violence occurs. The course of events after mass shootings, for example, have become frustratingly predictable. There follows a debate about which policy direction should be taken and it normally comes down to a binary choice—controlling the access to firearms (in a variety of different forms) or providing better prevention and treatment protocols involving mental health (in a manner that is very vaguely defined). Neither approach is ever adopted, and the issue normally is not brought up until the next highly publicized mass shooting occurs. It leaves many people in frustration, awaiting the next event with no action having been taken since the last one.

Suicide is another issue that garners attention around the issue of mental health. Though the exact extent of mental illness in completed suicides is unknown, it is certainly a potential contributor (Insel, 2011). Suicide is a leading cause of death nationally with several risk factors including depression and substance use disorders. The persons committing suicide are not the only ones affected—the traumatic effects are extended to family and friends of the deceased (CDC, 2015). Another worrisome fact is how it affects younger people; nearly 6,000 people died by suicide in 2015 (National Institute of Mental Health, 2018). It is often celebrity suicides, however, that bring the matter to national consciousness.

Writing in the years just prior to America's entrance into World War II, Pitirim Sorokin (1941) described the "crisis of our age" as a series of consequences resulting from periods of great transition, consequences that include increasing amounts of "mental disease" and higher rates of suicide. He contended that "the indispensable prerequisite of a sound and integrated mind is the presence of social stability and unchallenged general norms (1941, p. 207). He described, in much the same fashion as Durkheim (1897/1951)—that moral breakdown leads to mental illness and suicide, and that involvement with others is an antidote to these problems. Although concerns of a breakdown of society are probably unfounded, it is advantageous to take inventory of our current condition (not only from a personal but societal perspective) to analyze where we are and where we need to be. Recent sociological theorizing into the national character can be illustrative.

Global Risk and Instability

Ulrich Beck (1992) conceived of the idea of a "risk society" to define the crisis of our present age. This risk society, also described by other scholars, takes into factors such as how globalization at the micro level affects our individual lives. Beck referred to "new global risks" as catastrophic events that are created by humans (not nature) at a global level that negatively effects well-being. We can think of how many things put us at risk such as climate change, pollution, food toxicity, and large scale financial problems, such as the recent Great Recession. Current fears over nuclear war, for example, create existential threats to individual mental health. Also, the political divide currently evident around the world and nationally creates deep anxiety for many global citizens. Terrorism and other forms of violence, enduring concerns in present day society, also contribute to increased fear and anxiety. Global poverty, the lack of clean water, and various other conditions are also risk factors in modern society.

Another view of modern culture was shared by Zygmunt Bauman, who saw society as being in a state called "liquid modernity" (Bauman, 2000), which is marked by uncertainty and "conditions under which its members act change faster than it takes the ways of acting to consolidate into habit and routines" (Bauman 2005, p. 1). This new world is unpredictable, precarious, and uncertain, as humans constantly change to adapt to the conditions created by globalization, industrialization, and other facets of modernization. Individuality is compromised in this unstable, liquid existence and when we seek solution in mental health treatment in these times we find many "self-proclaimed helpers who (at the right price, of course) will be all too willing to guide us into the dark dungeons of our souls where our authentic selves are supposed to stay imprisoned and from where they are struggling to escape into the light" (Bauman 2005, p. 7). Bauman suggests however that this "movement into the light" does not slow the growth of our emotional troubles—it increases it. Loss of individuality is a cost of living in liquid modern times.

The world has also changed due to technology, especially in the form of electronic communications such as email, text, and messaging through social media. Due to changes in these areas, we have connected online but disconnected in face-to-face relationships. Online communication offers promise in some respects, but our "networked life allows us to hide from each other, even as we are tethered to each other" (Turkel 2011, p. 1). Studies show our connectivity simply leaves us feeling detached from society—the "elephant in the room is loneliness" (Olds and Schwartz 2009:5). Although human connectivity is a social issue, it is potentially psychological/biological as our brains are hard-wired to connect with other people (Liebermann, 2013). Alienation, isolation, exclusion, and basic devaluation of people (called "social undermining") all contribute to feelings of malaise and anxiety that contribute to mental distress (Oetzel, Duran,

Yizhou, & Lucero, 2007). As Perry (1974, p. 2) stated, "no one is more isolated than when withdrawn in an altered state of consciousness."

Whether the world is perceived as unstable by a series of human-made risks, a state of constant flux and instability, or the disconnect that comes from relying on electronic communication, the effects of these global and technological conditions on individual mental health are certain. The sociological imagination contains the essence of this relationship between personal biography and social history.

Structural Problems on a National Level

Problems at the national level, like those on the global scale, affect our emotional lives. America's structural inequality (like those in many other nations) exists in many forms, in race/ethnicity, sex/gender, class, age, and many others. These inequalities have long been observed by sociologists and are important in understanding the effects of these structural problems on mental health.

American mental health systems adapted through history to legitimize certain types of prejudice and discrimination. For example, a particularly repelling historical example of how the mental health system treated racial minorities was the establishment of a medical condition known as drapetomania that was determined to be a disorder affecting African slaves who fled from the slave holders—the "treatment", predictably, consisted of beatings. Women's experiences have also been subjected to stereotyping and medicalization as many "disorders" have been tailor-made for them such as nymphomania, hysteria, and currently, the "mental disorder" known as premenstrual dysphoric disorder. Neurasthenia was a diagnosis that came to be related to the upper class in society to explain the fatigue and stress resulting from living in high society—a disorder for the elites. Other conditions, such as transvestic disorder, which refers to sexual arousal from cross dressing, and gender dysphoria, the incongruence between assigned and experienced gender, also come into conflict with current ideas on gender and identity.

So, we continue in a perpetual state of distress. Sociologists, psychologists, and scholars from other disciplines provide research and theorize. Practitioners apply what is known about provision of services, however, this is done with political and economic realities contributing heavily to mental health practice. It appears our society is impotent in alleviating distress among a large population of our citizens. Where we are currently does not seem to be a great place—it is better than the past, but certainly not as good as we should imagine. Or reimagine.

By examining our current condition through the lens of history and by examining the various elements of our mental health system, including practices and policies, and by advocating for better conditions, we will put our reimagining to use. Conversations must occur directed toward this end.

WHERE WE HAVE BEEN: THE LENS OF HISTORY

In this book, we have used the history of mental health as a beacon to show where we have been to help plot a map for the future. This history has some deeply disturbing aspects, others we might consider humorous, and still others that show deeply human attempts to assist people to live their lives more fully. The lack of scientific understanding of mental illness in the past created many unorthodox practices, but those led us eventually to where are now.

We have seen how the earliest explanations of mental illness have involved spiritual explanations, increasingly adding bits of scientific knowledge to the point where they included biological explanations. We have also seen how the evolving social treatment of the mentally ill progressed from allowing the mad to wander the streets and countryside, to placing them in poorhouses and jails, to housing them in asylums, to releasing them when the asylums became warehouses for large numbers of mental patients. We have seen how communities were ill-equipped to adequately handle the effects of deinstitutionalization, as funding never supported this massive project.

Since most mentally ill people came to be seen in outpatient settings, a large variety of treatment modalities arose. The system itself was subsumed under the medical model as reflected not only in treatment methods but the assessment process and primary diagnostic instrument, the DSM series. War increased the need for mental health providers and psychiatrists were joined by psychologists and social workers, and later, marriage and family therapists, mental health nurses, and counselors, each having a treatment emphasis that differs in focus (sometimes slightly in practice, however) from the others.

Despite a sketchy history of the treatment of the mentally ill, a diverse group of advocates—from those who promoted moral treatment, advocated for greater mental hygiene, pushed for addiction recovery, and advocated other projects—have attempted to improve the conditions for the mentally ill and to better the mental health system. The issue of stigma has always followed those considered to be mentally disordered as they have always, to varying degrees, been ostracized and "othered".

It is beneficial to view the history of the treatment of the mentally ill and use this information to guide our efforts as we move through the next phases. President John F. Kennedy's call to action in 1963's Community Health Act offered some clear objectives in a vision for mental health care in the United States:

- bestowal of deserved benefits to those with mental disorders
- prevention of the occurrence of mental illness when possible
- provision of continuing care after appropriate diagnosis
- improvements in the level of care in public and private hospitals
- release of large numbers of committed asylum residents to community programs
- creation of effective health, educational, and rehabilitation services (Frank & Glied, 2006)

Progress has been made toward most of these goals as the lives of the mentally ill have been dramatically improved since 1963 (Frank & Glied, 2006). However, even though Americans with mental illness have overcome many barriers since the Community Mental Health Act, to concede the work in advocating for the mentally ill is done would be premature. The mentally ill continue to suffer from stigma, prejudice, discrimination, and violence, among other issues. It is a social justice cause to work on their behalf.

HOW WE ENDED UP HERE: IMAGININGS

Perhaps taking a moment to reflect on how modern culture plays a role in the mental health system would be advisable (O'Brien & Crowhurst, 2013). It is true we can use technology to alter the course of traditional psychotherapy and this is, in fact, happening with the advent of internet-based therapy. And the change from more in-depth, insight-based therapies and client-centered modalities of treatment have given way to short-term therapies that are meant to evaluate the problem quickly and, using the highly structured DSM, address the problem quickly through an assortment of prefabricated options for treatment. This is all part of the process known as rationalization, which is worthy of deeper consideration.

The process of rationalization

This process explains how society is changing by evolving its institutions based on the control of output, time, and personnel; many programs follow this pattern even though they do not always provide a good fit. For example, it appears the mental health "industry" is taking on the characteristics of the exemplars of rationalization, fast food restaurants, (O'Brien & Crowhurst, 2013) by rapidly providing a needed commodity with lower costs and a standard menu of items from which to choose. The product can be delivered quickly so the customer can move on to other activities. This fast food metaphor was aptly described in the *McDonaldization of America* in which sociologist George Ritzer (2002) described how so many aspects of our existence have come to resemble the model adopted by fast food chains. Ritzer described the primary features of this model—efficiency, calculability, predictability, and the use of non-human technology. Therefore, fast food restaurants serve as a model for the use of the most efficient methods for rapid provision of goods; for the quantification and calculation of many business actions; for assurances the products that are sold and the behavior of employees are basically the same in all restaurants; and the use, when possible, of machines that require little calculation or other decision-making ability, in food preparation or presentation, by the employees. In other words, due to the consistent rational maneuvering of food preparation and delivery, costs are kept low and customers are provided with a fast, predictable product and dining (or ordering) experience.

However, many diners bemoan the quality of the food or the lack of ambience that is found in a traditional restaurant. Few people have probably offered (or received) a marriage proposal in a fast food restaurant. And people in business probably refrain from taking a client with potentially lucrative potential to this type of restaurant. Culturally, there is a difference. An additional note is provided—Ritzer offered several other aspects of modern life that have adopted this model such as fitness clubs, vision centers, automobile lube and brake shops, salons, and many others. Perhaps we can add another to this list.

Ritzer's McDonaldization thesis was based on Max Weber's (1905/2003) concept of rationality, which states that as society becomes more complex and bureaucratized, characteristics such as tradition, customs, spirituality, and family ties give way to action that consists of greater rational calculation and a more intricate structure. As we become a society of consumers, it is predictable that the term mental health "consumers" came to be used in lieu of the older terms "patients" or "clients".

It can be seen then that the adoption of the fast food model doesn't legitimately fit mental health service provision; to even state this is revealing the obvious. A fast food model might accommodate an active lifestyle such as ordering food "on the go", but is that analogous to people seeking mental health treatment? Does this model compromise the quality of therapy for the sake of rational calculation? Should there be a chain store model of mental health that meets the requirements of efficiency, calculability, and predictability? And what about the therapists—are they really needed, or can a robot or computer program perform the same function? If a social determination is made that human therapists (instead of machines) should provide therapy, doesn't rushing to find diagnoses and providing brief treatments from a preformed planning guide basically result in "micromanaging" their time, thwarting their ability to pause and reflect on the client's presenting problems (O'Brien & Crowhurst, 2013)?

There are other issues of rationalization that take place in the mental health field. For example, professional licensure of practitioners and the professional accreditation of programs can be a convoluted and lengthy process but necessary to ensure the quality of care provided by people and programs meet certain standards; the term "best practices" is an attempt to condense standards to a concise practice model. The diagnostic process, as rationalized in the DSM, and therapeutic intervention, as rationalized in the continuing use of brief treatment modalities, are also evident. In addition, research in the mental health field, with its evolving methodologies, constitutes evidence of the increasing rationalization of field.

Psychotherapists have at their disposal many different "treatment planners" that address every conceivable condition and disorder; these treatment planners are basically like cookbooks that provide recipes for a chocolate cake. In a way these adopt the same modus operandi as the DSM—a ready guide to fit a problem. It makes the treatment process flow much faster. It also requires less skill and training of therapists. In short, it is less human.

Of special note in this rationalization process is the role of technology. Technology has long been a concern of societies. While it holds the potential to assist people in making systems, (such as the mental health system) more efficient and effective, it also carries some major drawbacks dealing with privacy concerns and the lack of face-to-face human contact which could add to a lack of humanity in the therapy process. Like the mythical John Henry fighting a new-fangled machine, there is always an underlying fear that the machine will win, taking our lives in the process. Technology can certainly enrich our lives and improve health care. But it does so at the risk of some important negative consequences. In 2017, a drug was approved for people with schizophrenia that includes a sensor that tracks if the drug was taken; when the pill is dissolved by the stomach fluids a message is relayed to a mobile app via a wearable patch, alerting medical health professionals that the pill was indeed swallowed (Brooks, 2017). While this certainly helps to ensure that patients are compliant in taking their medications, it also raises questions about the invasiveness of surveillance that takes place—in this case *within* the human body. The sociological concept of cultural lag posits that often one part of a culture, such as technology, progresses faster than the time it takes for a society's value system to accept the consequences of that technology, and can lead to a slowing of technological acceptance. On the other hand, certain technology-based therapeutic delivery systems such as video conversations between therapist and patient can potentially solve problems for homebound or remotely located patients.

History shows us that throughout human existence we have "understood" what was earlier termed madness in many ways—from supernatural occurrences, to acts of deviance, and currently as medical problems. We continue to imagine and reimagine mental illness. Imaginings have guided the stages that were mentioned in the chapter on history (from colonial times to the current focus on criminalization of the mentally ill) as American society has tried to correct and renegotiate those areas that have failed to fulfill their vision or that changed due to external conditions.

We currently place conditions connected with mental distress in the medical model. There are voices that accept and validate the primacy of psychiatry and the medical model while there are others that offer strong critiques. While acknowledging that psychiatry has long been the medical field's "awkward offspring" (p. 25), with its share of charlatanism, Lieberman (2015) extols the virtues and potentialities of both psychiatry and the DSM-5, which he dubbed the "unbridled triumph of pluralism" (p. 290). Psychiatry, he states,

> "...acquired the scientific knowledge and clinical capability to manage mental illness effectively and is attracting some of the best and the brightest talent into the profession, changing popular culture and society's attitudes toward psychiatry and mental illness has become the final, and perhaps most challenging, task of all."

Psychiatry in this light, then, is the vehicle to bring about positive change—if perceptions about it change.

Kelly (2009) also supports the medical model and believes the way to fix the system is to focus on results-oriented and evidence-based practices to create more competition between providers by removal of the monopoly of state systems, provision of insurance parity, empowerment of mental health consumers and the disbandment of the status quo. This position, progressive in the sense that engagement and empowerment will promote change, envisions the perceived curative powers of the free market as a change creator. In his view, positive change comes about by the mental health system changing to reflect capitalism rather than any internal changes in the system itself.

WHERE WE SHOULD BE: REIMAGININGS

While advocating the maintenance of psychiatry's prominence in the field of mental health and of the continued use of the medical model, Lieberman (2015) legitimately comments that "mental disorders represent a form of medical illness unlike any others" (p. 289). This is certainly true—they are very different, therefore, one might ask "why" those conditions considered mental disorders are considered medical conditions at all. We will return to this idea shortly.

Cohen (2016) casts a critical eye on a system which he posits supports a view of mental illness that is fundamentally flawed. His contention that so-called mental disorders do not fit the medical model for several reasons, including the fact that there exists no medical test that determines mental illness, there is no definitive correlation of mental illness to biological etiology, there is no successful treatment measure that is associated with an individual disorder, and there is no way to accurately predict outcomes of future cases. The dominance of psychiatry, according to Cohen (which he calls "psychiatric hegemony"), which includes psychopharmacology interventions, has resulted in a system of authority, enforced by neoliberalism, that other psy-professionals have bought into to preserve their own roles in society, thereby maintaining their own professional status. Less optimistic about the positive effects of minor change than Liebermann and Kelly, Cohen sees the only logical course as disrupting the current discourse by creating coalitions of academics, activists, community organizations, and survivor groups to advocate:

- removal of the compulsory powers of the psychiatric profession (such as involuntary commitment to institutions, invasive treatment measures, and forced drug ingestion)
- elimination of the prescribing rights of psychiatrists
- placement of accurate warning labels on prescribed medications
- illegalization of ECT procedures

Kinderman (2014) also rejects the use of the medical model in the mental health system and the disease model upon which it is derived. The use of this model creates conditions where psy-professionals fail to empathize with distressed people (he chooses not to use the term "patient") as the professionals begin to see them as carriers of disease rather than people who have been people dealing with various environmental stressors. Seeing the result of these stressors as a disease is an outdated approach; Kinderman uses pregnancy as an analogy—while there are a host of medical practitioners of different specialties that assist pregnant women, and there always exist possibilities that medical complications may occur during the pregnancy, pregnancy is not a disease.

Kinderman has provided a "manifesto for the reform of mental health and well-being services" (2014, p. 186) in which he outlines 8 provisions he believes will create a better system:

1. Abandonment of the disease model and replacement with a psychosocial model that treats people with psychological and social support rather than treatment of disease
2. Replacement of mental health diagnosis based on the medical model with a simple listing of problems encountered by the person
3. Reduction of the use of drugs by prescribing short-term use and when appropriate, replacement with other alternatives
4. Tailoring of treatment to individuals and abolishment of standardized treatment protocols
5. Rejection of coercive decisions and treatment and replacement with personal agency, except where harm to self or others might exist
6. Establishment of a multidisciplinary team with democratic values that accepts input from, but not an oversight by, psychiatrists
7. Community-based service provision, even in residential programs
8. Promotion of a broad program of wellbeing and health that includes social justice measures to combat discrimination of and abuse of vulnerable populations

Ferguson (2017) adopts a Marxist framework to describe how economic conditions create distressful responses in the working classes. Expressing that the current situation of mental health is a key issue of the current century, created and exacerbated by a capitalist system that alienates many people in occupational, educational, and family institutions. This alienation is a result of workers having no control over the product of their labor or the labor process itself, resulting in a disconnect in relating to others. Alienation contributes to mental distress through feelings of powerlessness and a loss of control—this distress has been medicalized and promoted by the drug industry.

Ferguson's ideas harken back to those of Friedrich Engels (1845/1987) who, in the mid-nineteenth century, chronicled the many negative consequences of worker exploitation in British factories of the era. Included among those consequences were health problems that come from living and working in squalid conditions; he also mentioned mental distress such as "a more or less hypochondriac, melancholy, irritable, nervous condition" (p. 138). Intemperance (addiction to alcohol) was another prominent consequence as downtrodden workers sought solace in the "public house". Even in this early period, Engels noted the influence of medication for "all conceivable ailments: Morrison's Pills, Parr's Life Pills, Dr. Mainwaring's Pills, and a thousand other pills, essences, and balsams, all of which have the property of curing all the ills that flesh is heir to" (Engels 1845/1987, p. 135). One such medication was an opiate solution (laudanum) called Godfrey's Cordial that caused addiction and death, especially in women and small children. Engels' reference to "quack remedies" employed by "cheap charlatans" anticipated the anti-psychiatry movement by over a century.

In referring to the recent focus on "recovery" in the mental health field, Ferguson (2017) recognizes the inspirational quality of increased independence and self-reliance of the mentally distressed but is concerned this emphasis can be used by those in power to limit services to them. Programs that provide collective power are instead recommended. The concept of recovery has deep roots in the medical model and should be excluded from the new paradigm.

Based on the suppositions by the "reimaginers" in this section: that the medical ("disease") model does not adequately fit problems of emotional distress; that psychiatry, which supports the medical model should therefore not retain its primacy; that the current diagnostic process is inadequate; and that treatment protocols should be changed to reflect social factors, we should consider these suggestions in our reimaginings.

Reimagining a better conceptualization of mental health and illness

First, a reimagining must occur regarding what constitutes our understandings of mental health and mental illness. Mental health suggests a functional condition that consists of a biological etiology (at least primarily), and mental illness as a deviation from the healthy condition, a condition that requires a medical assessment and medically oriented treatment protocols (which do include psychotherapy in many cases). The term "behavioral health" is imprecise since more than just behaviors are involved in mental health and since someone experiencing problems with behavioral health would be said to have a "behavioral illness"; the term behavioral health in this setting just seems to further medicalize human behaviors. In lieu of the concept of mental health, the term well-being has been used and instead of mental illness, distress seems more appropriate. Well-being is a term that implies a holistic perspective—that there are many elements of emotional comfort. Distress is a common term and is versatile enough to equate ideas at the global level (reflecting the risk society) as well as the community, family, and individual levels.

Reimagining the process of diagnosis and assessment

Regarding diagnosis and the DSM, there is much discussion of which disorders, if any, should be considered mental disorders—some say all while others say none, and there are others who say only the more biologically oriented disorders should be considered a mental illness. This seems to miss the point, however; there should be two categories here—physical disorders and "something else". The conditions that seem (at least currently) to have biological origins and that respond to medication, e.g., schizophrenia and bipolar disorder, should simply be considered disorders or illnesses, not *mental* disorders or *mental* illnesses. Those that are "something else", i.e., most of the others designated in the DSM such as personality disorders, anxiety disorders, and others, should be separately designated. Sleep disorders and other obvious medical disorders should also be considered health conditions. The conditions that are the "something else" should be labeled in a way to prevent the stigma of mental illness. As previously mentioned, the term often used by people of the non-medical camp is distress, though other terms could be used; anxiety is too closely related to the medical model at this point to distinguish the new paradigm.

Reimagining the provision of treatment services

The use of treatment teams is highly recommended with several professionals represented such as psychiatrists, psychologists, social workers, family therapists and counselors of different types. Sociologists have traditionally been excluded from any aspects of psychiatry; for example, in the DSM-5 fourteen groups are listed as contributors or consultants—not included are sociologists (one can surmise why this is the case). Sociologists are needed to provide understanding about how social stressors contribute to individual distress—notably poverty, unemployment, political discord (at local, state, and national levels), climate change, fears of war and violence, among other aspects inherent in the risk society—which should be at the heart of mental health care. Sociologists seek to find underlying patterns and arrangements that call into question the status quo and dig beneath the surface to reveal those hidden problems that need to be unearthed and analyzed. Psychiatry has long dominated the field of mental health, but it is time to closely observe the reasons behind maintaining the status quo and begin to make changes. A medical perspective is needed in many cases and psychiatrists should be part of the team, but not the leaders (at least in all cases).

Since the roots of most forms of what we consider mental illness are social in nature, it seems prudent to have social networks for people dealing with these issues. Support teams who meet in structured formats in the same vein as group therapy should be a standard form of treatment. Overseen by the treatment team mentioned above, therapy then becomes a social process, resulting in inclusion and acceptance rather than exclusion, alienation, and social undermining. Since most therapists are currently trained in individual therapy (except for family therapists and group therapists), this move will require some changes in the way graduate schools and programs train therapists. But it is a small price to pay.

Treatment protocols that rely on medications should be supervised closely and, as noted by Kinderman (2014), should be used no longer than is necessary or to any extent longer than what is needed. Medication has side effects and does not possess positive benefits for all sufferers. Alternative measures should be used whenever possible and the current focus on mindfulness provides notable options.

A Final Word

What is being sought is a change in how we reimagine the therapeutic substructure that underpins our current mental health system. A major question is how this will be financed. Changes in coverage will take a great deal of effort to sort out and put into practice. It is important that we prioritize correctly—after mass shooting events, many politicians claim we need to invest more in mental health. It has been almost two decades and many mass killings since the Columbine massacre in Colorado and mental health is still not a priority. It will fail to be a priority until we correctly conceptualize mental distress as a social disorder and find appropriate ways of dealing with it. Helping people with mental distress can, and should, be a priority and worthy of funding.

Those who believe that these measures mentioned above (or similar progressive initiatives) are impossible, should look back at how our mental system changed over time. This is why an understanding of history is so important and a major part of this book. Gone are the days when the mentally distressed were blistered, bled, leeched, spun, and dunked in water. Throughout history the system has changed and will continue to change—

the direction of this change is up to policy makers, who are influenced by reimaginers, who need to advocate for those in distress.

We will conclude this work with a list of organizations and contact info in the next, and final, chapter. The list is intended to assist consumers and their families with information on organizations that might assist them with various problems. The list also is intended for practitioners and others who are interested in the field, including those who wish to support and advocate for our neighbors who are experiencing mental distress. The time has come to envision a better system of mental health in America, and to make that vision a reality. And it is time for reimaginings of advocacy programs that adopt the changes listed in this book and/or other progressive programs that seek to provide relief to those suffering social distress.

Chapter 9

RESOURCES

This chapter provides a list of potential resources, active advocacy groups, and related information that can help people actively work toward change in the mental health system. The chapter offers contact information on governmental agencies and non-profit and not-for-profit organizations that will promote greater engagement in making decisions about the future of the system.

GOVERNMENTAL AGENCIES

Mentalhealth.gov

Contact Information:

Website Information: https://www.mentalhealth.gov/about-us.html

Address: 200 Independence Avenue, S.W. Washington, D.C. 20201

Organization Information:

mentalhealth.gov is a resource which is considered a one stop shop for people to become educated about mental health. This site can be helpful to explain what a mental health problem might look like and how to help someone with concerning symptoms. People who are dealing with mental health problems can also go here for support and resources. The website has assistance in 15 different languages and is extremely user friendly.

National Institute of Mental Health (NIMH)

Contact Information:

Website: https://www.nimh.nih.gov/about/index.shtml

Address: 6001 Executive Blvd, Rockville, MD 20852

Phone:

Press Office: 301-443-4536

National Suicide Prevention Lifeline: 1-800-273-8255

Organization Information:

The National Institute of Mental Health is one of 27 Institutes that create the National Institutes of Health. The mission behind NIMH is to reconstruct how society understands and treats mental illness through research, prevention, recovery, and cure. The public can utilize this federal agency for education on an array of mental health topics, to find treatment and to learn more about outreach, research priorities, funding, labs at NIMH, and news events. Access is free, people interested can sign up for email updates and there are publications available in Spanish.

The Substance Abuse and Mental Health Services Administration (SAMSHA)

Contact Information:

Website Information: https://www.samhsa.gov

Address: 5600 Fishers Lane Rockville, MD 20857

Phone: (877-726-4727)

Organization Information:

SAMSHA, a government agency, works to advance public health efforts regarding mental health and the impact of substance abuse. SAMSHA provides access to educational materials, assists users in finding help and treatment, partners with countless other agencies to create a cohesive system and opens communication about mental illness and substance abuse.

ADVOCACY ORGANIZATIONS, GENERAL

Active Minds

Contact Information:

Website: www.activeminds.org

Find your student chapter: http://www.activeminds.org/get-involved/student-chapters

Other ways to get involved: http://www.activeminds.org/get-involved

Organization Information:

Active Minds is a nonprofit which helps students on college campuses to speak openly about mental health. The organization has 433 chapters which are student run and focus on educating students about mental health awareness, empowering students to seek help and providing information on where help can be found. Visit their website to get involved in removing the stigma surrounding mental health and help create a comfortable environment.

Aunt Bertha

Contact Information:

Website: https://www.auntbertha.com

Website Support: https://auntbertha.zendesk.com/hc/en-us

Organization Information:

The main mission of Aunt Bertha is to connect people and programs. This comprehensive search platform can help people access care in their area if they need assistance with food, housing, education and health. In addition to thousands of other potential supports, people can search in their area for emergency mental health care, inpatient and outpatient care, and therapists as well other helpful resources for mental health.

American Foundation for Suicide Prevention (AFSP)

Contact Information:

Website: https://afsp.org

To get Involved: https://afsp.org/take-action/

To find Support: https://afsp.org/find-support/

Organization Information:

The American Foundation for Suicide Prevention works to support those affected by suicide, suicide survivors, and suicide attempt survivors. AFSP funds scientific research, educates the public about mental health and suicide prevention and supporting those dealing with the impacts of suicide. These efforts help create an open culture and remove stigmas about mental health and suicide.

Crisis Text Line

Contact Information:

Website: https://www.crisistextline.org

How to become a volunteer: https://www.crisistextline.org/volunteer/

Organization Information:

Crisis Text Line is a nonprofit organization changing the way people in crisis get help. This organization provides 24/7 confidential text support to anyone in crisis and is free to most phone carriers. Crisis Text Line utilizes data and collaboration to best support those in need via the use of text messaging and technology. People experiencing a crisis can text 741-741 to talk with a trained crisis counselor.

Daily Strength

Contact Information:

Website: https://www.dailystrength.org

Contact and support: https://support.dailystrength.org/hc/en-us/requests/new

Organization Information:

Daily Strength is a Sharecare company which provides support groups in a variety of areas including depression, PTSD, and anxiety. Users can select a support group, create their own posts, comment on posts, and connect with others experiencing similar struggles.

Find Your Words

Contact Information:

Website: https://findyourwords.org

Organization Information:

Find Your Words provides information on understanding depression, what to do if you want to support someone else or yourself if you are feeling depressed. The website also provides a self-assessment for users, as well as access to support and needed help. The website is also available in Spanish.

Half of Us

Contact Information:

Website: http://www.halfofus.com

Email: press@halfofus.com

Organization Information:

Half of Us is an advocacy group that has partnered with a few other groups including mtvU and The Jed Foundation to raise awareness and open public dialog regarding the prevalence of mental health issues and connect people with the proper resources.

Mental Health America (MHA)

Contact Information:

Find MHA in your area: http://www.mentalhealthamerica.net/find-affiliate

Contact: http://www.mentalhealthamerica.net/contact-us

Organization Information:

Mental Health America is a leading nonprofit in promoting the wellbeing of those living with mental illness and assisting in identification and connecting with services and supports. MHA is committed to educating the public about mental health, advocating for changes in policy and advocating connections between organizations to best help those dealing with mental health issues.

The Mighty

Contact Information:

Website information: HTTPs://themighty.com

Email: community@themighty.com or megan@themighty.com

Guidelines for material submission: https://themighty.com/submit-a-story/

Organization Information:

The Mighty is a website designed for people, by people and about people. The goal is to help those dealing with disease, disorder and disability and features thousands of articles written by people with experience in all those topics and more. Readers can submit articles and can read about real life accounts of mental illness.

To Write Love on Her Arms (TWLOHA)

Contact Information:

Website Information: https://twloha.com

Get Involved: https://twloha.com/get-involved/

Organization Information:

To Write Love On Her Arms is a nonprofit organization founded by someone who saw and felt the effects of mental illness, addiction, self-harm, and suicide first hand. Started to help a friend has turned into helping millions of people on their journey dealing with mental health. The main goal is to help those struggling with their mental health, create connections, informing and inspiring for treatment and recovery.

United Way and 211.org

Contact Information:

Website: www.unitedway.org

Website: http://211.org

Organization Information:

United Way is an organization whose mission is to bridge the gaps between health, education and financial stability in communities. United Way has partnered with countless other companies and organizations to achieve this, namely 211 which people can use to find resources in their area including mental health resources.

ADVOCACY ORGANIZATIONS FOR SPECIFIC DISORDERS

Anxiety Disorders—these disorders include Separation Anxiety Disorder, Specific Phobia, Social Anxiety Disorder (previously called social phobia), Panic Disorder, Agoraphobia, and General Anxiety Disorder. All anxiety disorders have at their core disturbances resulting from fear and anxiety—fear refers to a reaction to a real or imagined threat while anxiety is the anticipation of such a threat.

Anxiety and Depression Association of America (ADAA)

Contact Information:

Website: https://adaa.org

Address: 8701 Georgia Ave., Suite #412 Silver Spring, MD 20910

Phone: 240-485-1001

Organization Information:

This organization is useful to the public and mental health professionals alike. People who would like information can search in the "Understand the Facts>Anxiety" tab to learn more about different types of anxiety, signs and symptoms, ways to get help, and ways to manage anxiety. Additionally, mental health professionals can use this website to find research, events and continued education options. All areas of the website are open to anyone and the website can be translated into over 50 different languages.

Bipolar and Related Disorders—Bipolar disorder (previously referred to as manic-depressive disorder to describe the alternating pattern of mania and depression) is represented in Bipolar I and Bipolar II, and Cyclothymic Disorder. In manic phases, people in these categories experience elevated mood, increased activity, euphoria, irritability, and flight of ideas; when in the depressed phase, people experience depressed mood, sadness, decreased energy, and feelings of hopelessness. The alternating phases create many disruptions for the sufferer and those around them.

Depression and Bipolar Support Alliance

Contact Information:

Website: http://www.dbsalliance.org/site/PageServer?pagename=home

Address: 55 E. Jackson Blvd, Suite 490 Chicago, Illinois 60604

Phone: (800) 826-3632

Organization Information:

The Depression and Bipolar Support Alliance provides access to specific resources for those experiencing the effects of bipolar disorders. The website has sections to find educational tools, wellness and treatment options, and peer support. In addition to the resources for people with Bipolar Disorders, there are also resources for friends or family members looking for information about the best way to help those with bipolar disorders.

Depressive Disorders—these are the mood disorders that represent sadness, emptiness, irritability and the physical and cognitive responses that are connected to these conditions. Included in this group are Major Depressive Disorder, Persistent Depressive Disorder (previously called Dysthymia), and Premenstrual Dysphoric Disorder; these disorders are separated by the duration of the illnesses, along with timing and their presumed causes.

Anxiety and Depression Association of America (AADA)

Contact Information:

Website Information: https://adaa.org

Address: 8701 Georgia Ave., Suite #412 Silver Spring, MD 20910

Phone: 240-485-1001

Organization Information:

The Anxiety and Depression Association of American can be useful to those suffering from depressions or people who would like to learn more about depression. Users can go to the "Understand the Facts>depression" tab to learn about different types of depression and ways to cope or be treated. They can also learn about ways to get more support, find professional help, and even find events to spread awareness about depression. Mental health professionals can also benefit from this association to serve as easy access to facts, events, and continued education in their field.

Dissociative Disorders—dissociative disorders are those in which people have a disruption in consciousness, perception, body representation, and memory. People with these illnesses may feel unconnected with reality, with themselves, with their surroundings, or with their pasts (in the form of amnesia). Examples are Dissociative Identity Disorder, Dissociative Amnesia, and Depersonalization/Derealization Disorder.

National Alliance on Mental Illness (NAMI)

Contact Information:

Website: https://www.nami.org/Learn-More/ Mental-Health-Conditions/ Dissociative- Disorders/Treatment

Helpline: (800) 950-NAMI

Email: info@nami.org

Organization Information:

NAMI is an extensive organization that advocates for mental health and all mental illness alike. On this section of their website, users can find information, symptoms, causes, diagnosis, causes and treatment options for many dissociative disorders including dissociative amnesia and dissociative identity disorder. Those interested can also find access to support, a help line and text line and NAMI events in each state.

Disruptive, Impulse-Control, and Conduct Disorders—these disorders involve impulse control behaviors, such as aggression and violence, that result in the violation of the rights of others. Examples are Oppositional Defiant Disorder, Intermittent Explosive Disorder, Conduct Disorder), Antisocial Personality Disorder, Pyromania (fire-setting), and Kleptomania (theft). These disorders often involve the criminal justice system due to their close connection with injury (physical or psychological) or destruction.

Society for Adolescent Health and Medicine (SAHM)

Contact Information:

Website: https://www.adolescenthealth.org/Topics-in-Adolescent-Health/Mental-Health/Resources/Disruptive,-Impulse-Control-and-Conduct-Disorders.aspx

Phone: (847) 686-2246

Organization Information:

SAHM is a place to find resources about a variety of things related to health and mental health. One thing that can be found is information about disruptive, impulse-control and conduct disorders. there are videos to learn more information as well as toolkits and a resource guide for oppositional defiant disorder.

Psychiatry Advisory

Contact Information:

Website: http://www.psychiatryadvisor.com/anxiety/ understanding-impulse-control-and-conduct-disorders/article/383763/

Email: editor.PsychiatryAdvisor@HaymarketMedia.com

Organization Information:

The Psychiatry Advisor is an all-encompassing website which covers information regarding many different disorders, medications, and news about the field. Users can find information to better understand impulse control and conduct disorders according to the DSM-5, causes of disorders such as these, treatment options, and some additional resources.

Elimination Disorders—these disorders include behaviors that involve the elimination of urine and fecal matter from the body in inappropriate ways and places. Often first manifest in childhood and adolescence, examples are Enuresis and Encopresis.

National Association of Pediatric Nurse Practitioners

Contact Information:

Website: http://www.dbmhresource.org/elimination-disorders.html

Organization Information:

This website provides facts, available articles, other resources, and some criteria for diagnosis of those experiencing the effects of elimination disorders including enuresis and encopresis. Users seeking information about these disorders should utilize the individual links for each disorder as well as the "resources" section to discover additional organizations and support.

Feeding and Eating Disorders—the disorders in this category all involve the emotional and psychological disturbances involved in the process of eating. Examples are Anorexia Nervosa, Bulimia Nervosa, Binge-Eating Disorder, Rumination Disorder, Avoidant/Restrictive Intake Disorder and Pica (which involves eating non-food items).

National Eating Disorders Association (NEDA)

Contact Information:

Website: https://www.nationaleatingdisorders.org//

Phone: Helpline (800) 931-2237

Organization Information:

The NEDA is a useful organization to help educate people about eating disorders and provide ways to get involved. Additionally, the website has many options of ways that people suffering from an eating or feeding disorder can get support, including their helpline, chatting with a Helpline volunteer or texting into Crisis Text Line.

National Association of Anorexia Nervosa and Associated Disorders (ANAD)

Contact Information:

Website: http://www.anad.org

Phone: (630) 577-1333

Email: hello@anad.org

Organization Information:

The ANAD works to provide access to information regarding different eating and feeding disorders. People can use the website to find facts, signs and symptoms, treatment and support options and a blog. Additionally, users can call the helpline at (630) 577-1330 if they need urgent help or support.

Gender Dysphoria—this section is dedicated exclusively to gender dysphoria and includes Gender Dysphoria and Other Specified- and Unspecified Gender Dysphoria. This condition addresses controversial transgender issues and refers to the discomfort and distress experienced by people who experience an incongruence between their expressed and assigned gender, especially if reassignment measures are unaccusable. The term gender dysphoria replaces the DSM-IV's use of gender identity disorder to note the problematic condition is the clinical issue rather than a person's identity.

The Trevor Project

Contact Information:

Website: https://www.thetrevorproject.org/#sm.0000gio2cbj0dfbix8y10qrbq15wi

Phone: 1-866-488-7386

Organization Information:

The Trevor Project is an organization to provide educational tools, support, and resources available to LGBT youth. There is a TrevorLifeline, TrevorChat, TrevorText, TrevorSpace and Trevor Support center. This website is an all-inclusive and all-encompassing resource.

National Center for Transgender Equality

Contact Information:

Website: https://transequality.org/about-transgender

Address: 1133 19th St NW Suite 302 Washington DC 20036

Phone: 202-642-4542

Email: ncte@transequality.org

Organization Information:

The National Center for Transgender Equality website provides easy access to information about current issues, an area to learn facts about transgender people, laws and rights, ways to get involved and educational materials. Users can also find other resources through this website.

Neurodevelopmental Disorders—these are the disorders that are usually manifest in childhood that have a neurological cause and that continue through the life span. Included in this large category are Intellectual Disabilities (previously referred to as developmental disorders), Communication Disorders, Autism Spectrum Disorder, Attention-Deficit/Hyperactivity Disorder (ADHD), Specific Learning Disorder, and Motor Disorders.

Healthy Place

Contact Information:

Website: https://www.healthyplace.com/neurodevelopmental-disorders/

Contact Form: https://www.healthyplace.com/form/1-healthyplace-contact-form/

Organization Information:

The Healthy Place website provides information regarding neurodevelopmental disorders. Users can find educational materials about disorders including ADHD, autism, communication disorders, and motor disorders, as well as many more. Each disorder category outlines what the disorder is, treatment options, facts, tips and articles about that specific disorder.

National Autism Association

Contact Information:

Website: http://nationalautismassociation.org

Address: One Park Avenue, Suite 1 Portsmouth, RI 02871

Phone: (401) 293-5551

Organization Information:

The National Autism Association provides extensive resources and information for children, families and adults who have experience with autism and related disorders. This website is also helpful because it addresses some of the unique obstacles that autism and related disorders may bring. Users can find educational materials about safety, facts and treatment options. In addition, the website has access to support groups and programs, and ways to get involved.

Neurocognitive Disorders—this section refers to disorders involving cognitive functioning due to biomedical causes. Included are Delirium, and a long list of Major or Mild Neurocognitive Disorders (resulting from Alzheimer's Disease, Lewy Bodies, Vascular Disease, HIV infection, Prion Disease, Parkinson's Disease, Huntington's Disease, or other medical condition).

Health Line

Contact:

Website information: https://www.healthline.com/health/organic-brain-syndrome

Address:

-San Francisco Office, 660 Third Street San Francisco, CA 94107

-New York Office, 40 West 25th Street, 5th Floor New York, NY 10010

Phone:

-San Francisco Office (415) 281-3100

-New York Office (917) 720-4400

Organization Information:

The Health Line can be used to find symptoms, causes, treatment and other educational tools regarding neurocognitive disorders. users can follow links for specific neurocognitive disorders including Alzheimer's, dementia, prion, and multiple sclerosis to learn more about each disorder individually. The website also has a symptom checker, a pill identifier, and a place to find online doctors. It should be noted that if users are concerned about their mental state or someone in their life, they should seek professional medical attention.

Obsessive-Compulsive and Related Disorders—the disorders in which the sufferer has obsessions (thoughts or urges that are persistent and troubling that a person consistently ponders) and compulsions (behaviors that are persistently performed to relieve the obsessive thought patterns). Included in this category are Obsessive-Compulsive Disorder (often referred to by its initials OCD), Body Dysmorphic Disorder, the newly added

Hoarding Disorder, Trichotillomania (hair pulling), and Excoriation (skin-picking).

International OCD Foundation

Contact Information:

Website: https://iocdf.org

Phone: (617) 973-5801

Email: info@iocdf.org

Organization Information:

The International OCD Foundation works to raise awareness about OCD and related disorders. The Foundation provides access to effective treatment options, educational materials, ways to help or donate and namely helps to break down stigmas against mental illness which users can also learn about on their website.

Personality Disorders—the group of disorders is characterized by personality traits that are inflexible and maladaptive and that generate behaviors that deviate sharply from the person's cultural norms. There are many disorders in this grouping that have varying characteristics, manifestations, and symptoms. Included in this category are Antisocial Personality Disorder, Borderline Personality Disorder, Narcissistic Personality Disorder, Histrionic Personality Disorder, and Schizoid Personality Disorder.

Personality Disorders Awareness Network

Contact Information:

Website: http://www.pdan.org

Phone: (937) 732-9273

Address: 1072 W Peachtree St. NW, #79468 Atlanta, GA 30357

Email: info@pdan.org

Organization Information

The Personality Disorders Awareness Network is an all-encompassing non-profit focusing on educating the public about personality disorders. the website has extensive educational tools about different disorders including borderline and antisocial, users can find statistics and facts. In addition to the education portion, users can find programs, additional resources, and a blog.

Paraphilic Disorders—these disorders involve sexual behavior often considered deviant that contain harmful or potentially harmful consequences to others. Included are Voyeuristic Disorder, Exhibitionistic Disorder, Frotteuristic Disorder, Sexual Masochism Disorder, Sexual Sadism Disorder, Pedophilic Disorder, and Fetishistic Disorder. These disorders are closely tied with the criminal justice system as others are often harmed in the commission of paraphilic behaviors.

Mental Health Learning Center

Contact Information:

Website: http://www.mentalhealthlearningcenter.org/index.php/paraphilic-disorders

Organization Information:

This website is a useful tool to help become educated about different paraphilic disorders. Those who are experiencing the effects of disorders such as exhibitionistic, fetishistic, paraphilic, and pedophilic disorders or anyone who would like more information can find possible resources in the community and different options for treatment.

Schizophrenia Spectrum and other Psychotic Disorders—these are the disorders with psychotic features and involve delusions, hallucinations (visual, audial, or other sensory modality) disordered thinking, and disorganized motor activity. Disorders such as Schizophrenia, Schizotypal Disorder, Schizoaffective Disorder, Catatonia, and Delusional Disorder are part of this spectrum. Note—the idea of a spectrum suggests a continuum of characteristics and related symptomology.

Schizophrenia and Related Disorders Alliance of America

Contact Information

Website: https://sardaa.org

Phone: 240-423-9432

Address: P.O Box 941222 Houston, TX 77094

Email: info@sardaa.org

Organization Information:

SARDAA stands for Schizophrenia and Related Disorders Alliance of America. This organization focuses on the support, recovery, education, and advocacy of schizophrenia and related illnesses. Users can find extensive related resources, an educational blog, events, and peer support access on the website.

Sexual Dysfunctions—these include problems in sexual activity and deals with the psychological effect of conditions that inhibit a person's ability to respond to or enjoy sexuality; in this section are Delayed Ejaculation, Erectile Disorder, and Female Orgasmic Disorder.

Cleveland Clinic

Contact Information:

Website: https://my.clevelandclinic.org/health/articles/an-overview-of-sexual-dysfunction

Phone:

Appointments: (866)-320-4573

Questions: (800) 223-2273

Organization Information:

The Overview of Sexual Dysfunction on the Cleveland Clinic website is a useful resource to provide information about sexual dysfunction. People can find facts and types, who may be affected, symptoms, diagnosis and possible treatment options. Additionally, users can request an appointment online and find additional contact information for doctors if they are interested.

Sleep-Wake Disorders—these disorders include the ways in which inappropriate sleep patterns (involving quality, timing, and amount) can cause psychological issues. These conditions include Insomnia Disorder, Narcolepsy, Obstructive Sleep Apnea, Sleep-Related Hypoventilation, and Circadian Rhythm Sleep-Wake Disorders.

Sleep Education

Contact Information:

Website: http://sleepeducation.org

Phone: (630) 737-9700

Address: 2510 North Frontage Road, Darien, IL 60561

Organization Information:

The Sleep Education website provided by the American Academy of Sleep Medicine can be used to find educational material about numerous sleep-wake disorders. Users can find symptoms, treatment options, and facts about a disorder they may be facing. Additionally, users can search for a sleep center in their area which could be a possible treatment for them.

Somatic Symptom and Related Disorders—these are emotional disorders that reflect physical conditions in which the people suffering from them are primarily seen in medical settings such as primary care institutions rather than mental health establishments. Examples include Somatic Symptom Disorder, Illness Anxiety Disorder, and Conversion Disorder.

Mayo Clinic-Somatic Symptom Disorder

Contact Information:

Website: https://www.mayoclinic.org/diseases-conditions/somatic-symptom-disorder/symptoms-causes/syc-20377776

Phone: (480) 301-8000

Organization Information:

The Somatic Symptom Disorder of the Mayo Clinic website can be used to learn more about what somatic symptom disorders and related disorders are, signs and symptoms and when to see a doctor if someone is concerned. Those interested can also find causes, risk factors, and possible ways to prevent somatic symptom disorder or related disorders. Additionally, one can learn about diagnosis, criteria for diagnosis, and possible treatment options.

Trauma- and Stressor-Related Disorders—these disorders are related to the experience of a real or perceived threat creates stress and anxiety. These include Post-Traumatic Stress Disorder, Reactive Attachment Disorder, Reactive Attachment Disorder, Disinhibited Stress Engagement Disorder, Acute Stress Disorder, and Adjustment Disorders.

International Society for the Study of Trauma and Dissociation

Contact Information:

Website: http://www.isst-d.org

Phone: (703) 610-9037

Email: info@isst-d.org

Organization Information:

The International Society for the Study of Trauma and Dissociation is an all-encompassing resource for anyone who seeks more information about trauma and dissociation. There are different sections for students and professionals as well as an area to find information specifically regarding children and adolescents. Users can also learn about treating trauma and dissociative disorders, read journals and articles, and find a therapist through the website.

REFERENCES

Acker, C. J. (2002). *Creating the American junkie: Addiction research in the classical era of narcotic control.* Baltimore and London: Johns Hopkins University Press.

Altschule, M. D. (1977). *Origins of concepts of human behavior: Social and cultural factors.* New York: Halstead Press.

American Association of Marriage and Family Therapy. (n.d.). Retrieved from www.aamft.org.

American Counseling Association. (n.d.). Retrieved December 12, 2017, from www.counseling.org

American Heritage Dictionary of the English Language (4th ed.). (2000). Boston and New York: Houghton Mifflin Co.

American Psychiatric Association. (n.d.). Retrieved from www.psychiatry.org.

American Psychiatric Nurses Association. (n.d.). Retrieved from www.apna.org.

American Psychological Association. (n.d.). Retrieved from www.apa.org.

American Psychiatric Association. (2013). *Diagnostic and statistical manual of mental disorders* (5th ed.). Arlington, VA: American Psychiatric Publishing.

Anderson, R. E., & Carter, I. (1990). *Human behavior in the social environment: A social systems approach* (4th ed.). New York: Aldine de Gruyter.

Astramovich, R. L., & Hoskins, W. J. (2013). Evaluating addictions counseling programs: Promoting best practices, accountability, and advocacy. *Journal of Addictions and Offender Counseling 34*(2), 114-124. doi: 10.1002/j.2161-1874.2013.00019.x

Badley, K. (1996). *Worldviews: The challenge of choice.* Toronto: Irwin.

Barker, P. (1985). *Using metaphors in psychotherapy.* New York: Brunner/Mazel.

Barker, P. (1986). *Basic family therapy* (2nd ed.). New York: Oxford University Press.

Bauman, Z. (2000). *Liquid modernity.* Cambridge, UK: Polity Press.

Bauman, Z. (2005). *Liquid life.* Cambridge, UK: Polity Press.

Baumohl, J. (1990). Inebriate institutions in North America: 1840-1920. *British Journal of*

Addiction 85 (9), 1187-1204.

Beck, U. (1992). *Risk society: Toward a new modernity.* London: Sage.

Beers, C. W. (1935). *A mind that found itself: An autobiography.* Garden City, New York: Doubleday, Doran, and Company.

Bellah, R. N., Madsen, R., Sullivan, W. M., Swidler, A., & Tipton, S. M. (1985). *Habits of the heart: Individualism and commitment in American life.* New York: Harper and Row.

Berger, P. L., & Luckmann, T. (1966). *The social construction of reality.* Garden City, NY: Doubleday.

Berlim, M., Fleck, M. P.A., & Shorter, E. (2003). Notes of antipsychiatry. *European archives of psychiatry and clinical neuroscience 253,* 61-67. Retrieved from http://research.flagler.edu:9838/eds/pdfviewer/pdfviewer?vid=1&sid=33255904-1fa6-4829-b50e-e3ed2515b1a4%40pdc-v-sessmgr01.

Bertalanffy, L. (1968). *General system theory: Foundations, development, applications.* London: Penguin Books.

Bose, J., Hedden, S. L, Lapari, R. N., & Park-Lee, E. (2016). Key substance use indicators in the United States: Results from the 2015 national survey on drugs and health. *Substance Abuse Mental Health and Services Administration.* (HHS Publication No. SMA 16-4984, NSDUH Series H-51). Retrieved from https://www.samhsa.gov/data/sites/default/files/NSDUH-FFR1-2015/NSDUH-FFR1-2015/NSDUH-FFR1-2015.htm.

Bowen, E. A., & Walton, Q. L. (2015). Disparities and the social determinants of mental health and addictions: Opportunities for a multifaceted social work response. *Health 40*(3), e59-e75. doi: 10.1093/hsw/hlv034

Brandt, A. L. S. (2012). Treatment of persons with mental illness in the criminal justice system: A literature review. *Journal of offender rehabilitation 51*(8), 541-558.

Breggin, P. (1994). *Toxic Psychiatry: Why therapy, empathy, and love must replace the drugs, electroshock, and biochemical theories of the 'new psychiatry'.* New York: St. Martin's Press.

Brooks, J. (2017). Patient-compliance sensor pill approved for use in US. *Electronics weekly 2017.* Retrieved from http://research.flagler.edu:9839/eds/detail/detail?vid= 0&sid=6dfe0941-8921-4ad5-b96dc1ce782460ae%40sessionmgr4009&bdata=JnNpdGU9ZWRzLWxpdmUmc2NvcGU9c2l0ZQ%3d%3d#AN=126483472&db=buh.

Bromberg, W. (1959). *The mind of man: A history of psychotherapy and psychoanalysis.* New York: Harper Torchbooks.

Bronfenbrenner, U. (1977). Toward an experimental ecology of human development. *American psychologist 32*(7), 513-531

Brown, N. W. (2013). *Creative activities for group therapy.* New York and London: Routledge.

Buchman, D. Z., Leece, P., & Orkin, A. (2017). The epidemic of stigma: The bioethics of opioids. *The Journal of Law, Medicine, and Ethics, 45*(4), 607-620. doi: 10.1177/1073110517750600

Burgess, E. (1926). The family as a unit of interacting personalities. *The Family* 7(1), 3-9.

Burns, Tom. (2006). *Psychiatry: A Very Short Introduction.* Oxford, UK: Oxford University Press.

Busfield, J. (2000). Introduction: Rethinking the sociology of mental health. *Sociology of Health & Illness,* 22(5), 543-558. doi: 10.1111/1467-9566.00219

Calloway, E. (2007). *Asylum: A mid-century madhouse and its lessons about our mentally ill today.* Westport, CN: Praeger.

Carlson, L. A., & Kees, N. L. (2013). Mental health services in public schools: A preliminary study of school counselor perceptions. *Professional School Counseling 16*(4), 211-221. Retrieved from http://research.flagler.edu:9839/eds/pdfviewer/pdfviewer?vid=1&sid=f27080d2-0916-4598-ba2f-125bc2acd861%40sessionmgr4006

Carr, A., & McNulty, M. (2006). Cognitive behavior therapy. In A. Carr & M. McNulty (Eds.), *The handbook of adult clinical psychology: An evidence-based practice approach.* London and New York: Routledge.

Carter, R. (1999). *Helping someone with mental illness: A compassionate guide for family, friends, and caregivers.* New York: Three Rivers Press.

Castrol, D., & Fritchle, M. (2013). Working with the queer community: Advocacy as a therapeutic intervention. In D. Maller & K. Langsam (Eds.), *The Praeger handbook of community mental health practice* (pp. 67-83). Santa Barbara, CA; Denver, CO; and Oxford, England: Praeger.

Center for Disease Control and Prevention (CDC). (2015). Understanding suicide: Fact sheet. Retrieved from https://www.cdc.gov/violenceprevention/pdf/suicide_factsheet-a.pdf.

Centers for Disease Control (CDC). (n.d.) *Heroin overdose data.* Retrieved December from https://www.cdc.gov/drugoverdose/data/heroin.html.

Centers for Disease Control (CDC). (n.d.) *Prescription opioid overdose data.* Retrieved from https://www.cdc.gov/drugoverdose/data/overdose.html.

Chapman, A.L. (2006). Dialectic Behavior Therapy. *Psychiatry.* 3 (9) 62-68. Retrieved from https://www.ncbi.nlm.nih.gov/pmc/articles/PMC2963469/.

Chesler, P. (1972). *Women and madness.* Garden City, NY: Doubleday and Company.

Church, M. A., & Brooks, C. I. (2009). *Subtle suicide: Our silent epidemic of ambivalence about living.* Santa Barbara, CA; Denver, CO, and Oxford, England. Praeger.

Churchman, C. W. (1979). *The systems approach and its enemies.* New York: Basic Books.

Clegg, J. W. (2012). Teaching about mental health and illness through the history of the DSM. *History of Psychology, 15* (4), 364-370. doi: 10.1037/a0027249.

Cohen, B.M.Z. (2016). *Psychiatric hegemony: A Marxist theory of mental illness.* London: Macmillan.

Cooley, C. H. (1902). *Human nature and the social order.* New York: Charles Scribner's Sons.

Coontz, S. (1992). *The way we never were: American families and the nostalgia trap.* New York: BasicBooks.

Corrigan, P. W., & Kleinlein, P. (2005). The impact of mental illness on stigma. In P. Corrigan (Ed.), *On the stigma of mental illness* (pp. 11-44). Washington, DC: American Psychological Association.

Concalves, O. F., Machado, P. P. P., Korman, Y. & Angus, L. (2002). Assessing psychopathology: A narrative approach. In M. L. Malik and L. E. Beutler (Eds.),

Rethinking the DSM: A psychological perspective (149-176). Washington, DC: American Psychiatric Association.

Crown, S. (1975). On being sane in insane places: A comment from England. *Journal of Abnormal Psychology, 84*(5), 453-455.

Cutler, D. L., Sills, G. M., Svendsen, D., & Yeager, K. R. (2013). Public mental health in America: 'Enlightenment' to accountable care. In K. R. Yeager, D. L. Cutler, D. Svendsen, and G. M. Sills (Eds.), *Modern mental health: An interdisciplinary approach.* New York: Oxford University Press.

Davis, D. M., & Hayes, J. A. (2011). What are the benefits of mindfulness? A practice review of psychotherapy-related research. *Psychotherapy 48*(2), 198-208. Retrieved from http://research.flagler.edu:9839/eds/pdfviewer/pdfviewer?vid=1&sid=c94df459-fa82-4c1c-9078-dfe84e90daf7%40sessionmgr4009

Dembo, R. & Pacheco, K. (1999). Criminal justice responses to adolescent substance abuse. In R. T. Ammerman, P. J. Ott, and R. E. Tarter (Eds.),

Prevention and societal impact of drug and alcohol abuse. Mahwah, NJ and London: Lawrence Erlbaum Associates.

Dies, R. R. (2003). Group psychotherapies. In A. Carr & M. McNulty (Eds.), *The handbook of adult clinical psychology: An evidence-based practice approach.* London and New York: Routledge.

Deutsch, A. (1948). *The Shame of the states.* New York: Harcourt, Brace.

Deutsch, A. (1949). *The mentally ill in America: A history of their care and treatment from colonial times* (2nd ed.). New York: Columbia University Press.

Donigan, J., & Malnati, R. (1997). *Systemic group therapy: A triadic model.* Pacific Grove, CA: Brooks/Cole Publishing Co.

Drack, M., & Pouvreau, D. (2015). On the history of Ludwig von Bertalanffy's 'General Systemology' and on its relation to cybernetics—Part III: Convergences and divergences. *International Journal of General Systems 44*(5), 523-57. doi: 0.1080/03081079.2014.1000642

Dualdiagnosis.com. (2018). Acceptance and Commitment Therapy. Retrieved from https://www.dualdiagnosis.org/treatment-therapies-for-dual-diagnosis-patients/acceptance-commitment-therapy/.

Durkheim, E. (1897/1951). *Suicide: A Study in sociology.* G. Simpson (Ed. and Trans.) New York: Free Press.

Durkheim, E. (1909/1982). *The rules of sociological method.* Introduction and selection by S. Lukes (Ed.) and W.D. Halls (Trans.). New York: Free Press.

Ellis, A. (1978). Family therapy: A phenomenological and active-directive approach. *Journal of Marriage and Family Counseling.* 4, 43-50.

Engel, J. (2008). *American therapy: The rise of psychotherapy in the United States.* New York: Penguin.

Engels, F. (1845/1987). *The conditions of the working class in England.* London: Penguin Books.

Epstein, M. (1995). *Thoughts without a thinker: Psychotherapy from a Buddhist perspective.* New York: Basic Books.

Erickson, P. E., & Erickson, S. K. (2008). *Crime, punishment and mental illness: Law and the behavioral sciences in conflict.* New Brunswick, NJ and London: Rutgers University Press.

Fancher, R. T. (1995). *Cultures of healing: Correcting the image of American mental health care.* New York: W.H. Freeman and Company.

Fatayer, J. (2008). Addiction types: A clinical sociology perspective. *Journal of Applied Social Sciences, 2*(1), 88-93. Retrieved from http://research.flagler.edu:9101/openurlsid=EBSCO%3asih&genre=article&issn=19367244&ISBN=&volume=2&issue=&date=20080401&spage=88&pages=883&title=Journal+of+Applied+Social+Sciences+(19367244)&atitle=Addiction+Types%3a+A+Clinical+Sociology+Perspective.&aulast=Fatayer%2c+Jawad&id=DOI%3a&site=ftf-live.

Ferguson, I. (2017). *Politics of the mind: Marxism and mental distress.* London: Bookmarks.

Fletcher, A.M. (2013). *Inside rehab: The surprising truth about addiction treatment—and how to get help that works.* New York: Viking.

Foucault, M. (1988). *Madness and civilization: A history of insanity in the age of reason.* New York: Vintage Books.

Fox, A. B., Earnshaw, V. A., Taverna, E. C., & Vogt, D. (2017). Conceptualizing and measuring mental illness stigma: The mental illness stigma framework and critical review of measures. *Stigma and Health.* Online First Publication. Received February 12, 2018. https://www.researchgate.net/publication/319974991_Conceptualizing_and_Measuring_Mental_Illness_Stigma_The_Mental_Illness_Stigma_Framework_and_Critical_Review_of_Measures.

Frances, A. (2013). *Saving Normal: An insider's revolt against out-of-control psychiatric diagnosis, DSM-5, big pharma, and the medicalization of ordinary life.* New York: William Morrow.

Frank, R. G., & Glied, S. A. (2006). *Better but not well: Mental health policy in the United States since 1950.* Baltimore, MD: The Johns Hopkins University Press.

Frankena, W. K. (1962). The concept of social justice. In R. B. Brandt, *Social Justice.* Englewood Cliffs, NJ: Prentice-Hall.

Frederickson, J. (1999). *Psychodynamic psychotherapy: Learning to listen to multiple perspectives.* Philadelphia: Brunner/Mazel.

Fromm, E. (1941). *Escape from freedom.* New York: Avon Books.

Fromm, E. (1955). *The sane society.* New York: Henry Hold and Company.

Germer, C. K. (2013). Mindfulness: What is it? What does it matter? In C. K. Germer, R. A. Siegel, & P. R. Fulton (Eds.), *Mindfulness and psychotherapy* (2nd ed.). New York and London: The Guilford Press.

Gilman, C.P. (1892). The yellow wallpaper. *The New England Magazine* *11*(5), 647-657.

Gilman, C. P. (1913). Why I wrote the yellow wallpaper. *The Forerunner.* Retrieved from https://www.nlm.nih.gov/exhibition/theliteratureofprescription/education/materials/WhyIWroteYellowWallPaper.pdf

Goffman, E. (1961). *Asylums: Essays on the social situation of mental patients and other inmates.* New York: Anchor Books.

Goffman, E. (1963). *Stigma: Notes on the management of spoiled identity.* New York: Simon and Schuster.

Goldfield, D. R., & Brownell, B. A. (1979). *Urban America: From downtown to no town.* Boston: Houghton Mifflin Company.

Gouldner, A. W. (1970). *The coming crisis of Western sociology.* New York and London: Basic Books, Inc.

Gribben, A. (1972). Mark Twain, phrenology and the "temperaments": A study of pseudoscientific influence. *American Quarterly.* 24 (1), 45-68. Retrieved from http://research.flagler.edu:9017/stable/pdf/2711914.pdf

Grob, G. N. (1991). Origins of DSM-1: A study in appearance and reality. *American Journal of Psychiatry 148*(4), 421-431. doi: org/10.1176/ajp.148.4.421

Hajar, R. (2012). The air of history: Early medicine to Galen (part one). *Heart Views 13*(3), 120-128. doi: 10.4103/1995-705X.102164

Halleck, S. L. (1971). *The politics of therapy.* New York: Science House, Inc.

Hamachek, D. E. (1978). *Encounters with the self* (2nd ed.). New York: Holt, Rinehart, and Winston.

Hatzenbuehler, M. L. (2014). Introduction to the special issue on structural stigma. *Social Science and Medicine, 103,* 1-6. Retrieved from https://www.deepdyve.com/lp/elsevier/introduction-to-the-special-issue-on-structural-stigma-and-health-VvHsL7qlWJ.

Henderson, R. and Pochin, M. (2001). *A right result? Advocacy, justice and empowerment.* Bristol: Policy Press.

Hiday, V. A., & Burns, P. J. (2010). Mental illness and the criminal justice system. In T. L Scheid and T. N. Brown (Ed.). *A handbook for the study of mental health: Social contexts, themes, and subsystems.* New York: Cambridge University Press.

Hill, T. D., & Maimon, D. (2013). Neighborhood context and mental health. In C. S. Aneshensel, J. C. Phelan, & Alex Bierman, (Eds.), *Handbook of the sociology of mental health* (2nd ed.). New York and London: Springer.

Hilton, C. (2017). *Improving psychiatric care for older people: Barbara Robb's campaign 1965-1975* Basingstoke, United Kingdom: Palgrave MacMillan. doi: 10.1007/978-3-319-54813-5.

Hodge, J. G., Wetter, S. A., & Noe, S. A. (2017). Emerging legal responses to curb the opioid epidemic. *Journal of law, medicine, and ethics 45*(3), 460-463. doi: 10.1177/1073110517737547

Hoffman, B. (2012). *Health care for some: Rights and rationing in the United States since 1930.* Chicago and London: The University of Chicago Press.

Horkheimer, Max. (1947). *Eclipse of reason.* New York: Oxford University Press.

Horowitz, A.V. (2002). *Creating mental illness.* University of Chicago Press. Horowitz, A. V. (2010). An overview of sociological perspectives on the definitions, causes, and responses to mental health and illness. In T. Scheid and T. Brown (Eds.), *A handbook for the study of mental health: Social contexts, theories, and systems* (pp. 6-19) (2nd ed.). Cambridge: Cambridge University Press.

Houts, A. C. (2002). Discovery, invention, and the expansion of the modern diagnostic and statistical manuals of mental disorders. In L. E. Beutler and M. L. Malik (Eds.) *Rethinking the DSM: A Psychological Perspective.* Washington: American Psychological Association.

Hoyt, M. F. (2003). Brief Psychotherapies. In A. S. Gurman and S. B. Messer, *Essential psychotherapies: Theory and practice* (2nd ed.) (pp.350-399). New York and London: Guilford Press.

Insel, T. (2011). Post by former NIMH director Thomas Insel: Understanding severe Mental illness. Retrieved from https://www.nimh.nih.gov/about/directors/thomas-insel/blog/2011/understanding-severe-mental-illness.shtml.

Joffe, J. L. (2016). Don't call me crazy: A survey of America's mental health system. *Chicago-Kent Law Review 91*(3), 1145-1196. http://scholarship.kentlaw.iit.edu/cklawreview/vol91/iss3/12.

Jonas, S., Goldsteen, R. L., & Goldsteen, K. (2013). *Jonas' introduction to the U.S. health care system* (7th ed.). New York: Springer.

Johnson, A. B. (1990). *Out of Bedlam: The truth about deinstitutionalization.* New York: Basic Books.

Kelly, T. A. (2009). *Healing the broken mind: Transforming America's failed mental health system.* New York and London: New York University Press.

Kinderman, P. (2014). *A prescription for psychiatry: Why we need a whole new approach to mental health and wellbeing.* Basingstoke, Hampshire UK: Palgrave Macmillan.

Kirk, S.A. & Kutchins, H. (1992). *The selling of DSM: The rhetoric of science in psychiatry.* New York: Adline.

Kirk, S., Gomory, T., & Cohen, D. (2013). *Mad science: Psychiatric coercion, diagnosis, and drugs.* New Brunswick, NJ: Transaction Publishers.

Klein, R.H., Bernard, H. S., & Singer, D. L. (1992). Introduction. In R. H. Klein, H. S. Bernard, and D. L. Singer (Eds.), *Handbook of contemporary group psychotherapy* (pp.1-23). Madison, CN: International Universities Press.

Klenowski, P. M., Bell, K. J., & Dodson, K. D. (2010). An empirical evaluation of juvenile awareness programs in the United States: Can juveniles be "scared straight"? *Journal of Offender Rehabilitation 49*(3), 254-272. doi: 10.1080/10509671003716068

Kline, P. (1984). *Psychology and Freudian theory: An introduction.* London and New York: Methuen.

Kuhn, C., Swartzenwelder, S., and Wilson, W. (2008). *Buzzed: The straight facts about the most used and abused drugs from alcohol to ecstasy* (3rd ed.) New York and London: W. W. Norton and Company.

Kurtz, L. F. (1987). Historical perspectives on the care and treatment of the mentally ill. *The Journal of Sociology and Social Welfare 14* (4), 75-94.

Kushner, H. I. (1988). Beyond social construction: Toward new histories of psychiatry. *Journal of the history of the neurosciences, 7*(2), 141-149.

LaBruzza, A. L. (1997). *Using DSM-IV: A Clinician's guide to psychiatric diagnosis.* Northvale, NJ and London: Jason Aronson Inc.

Laing, A. (1994). *R.D. Laing: A biography.* New York: Thunder's Mouth Press.

Laing, R.D. (1960). *The divided self.* Tavistock: Penguin Books.

Lane, J. B. (2000). Overview of assessment and treatment issues. In M. Hersen & M. Biaggio, (Eds.), *Effective brief therapies* (pp.3-15). San Diego: Academic Press.

Larner, G., Strong, T. & Busch, R. (2013). Family therapy and the spectre of the DSM-5. *Australian and New Zealand Journal of Family Therapy, 34*(2), 87-89. doi: 10.1002/anzf.1013

Lasch, C. (1979). *The culture of narcissism: American life in an age of diminishing expectations.* New York: W.W. Norton.

Lemert, E. M. (1967). *Human deviance, social problems, and social control.* Englewood Cliffs, NJ: Prentice Hall.

Lender, M. E. & Martin, J. K. (1987). *Drinking in America: A history,* Revised and Expanded Edition. New York: The Free Press.

Levin, W. C. (1991). *Sociological ideas* (3rd ed.). Belmont, CA: Wadsworth Publishing Co. Levine, M. (1981). *The history and politics of community mental health.* New York and Oxford: Oxford University Press.

Lieberman, J. A. (2015). *Shrinks: The untold story of psychiatry.* New York, Boston, and London: Back Bay Books.

Liebermann, M. D. (2013). *Social: Why our brains are wired to connect.* New York: Broadway Books.

Link, B. G., & Phelan, J. C. (2001). Conceptualizing stigma. *Annual Review of Sociology 27,*363-385. Retrieved from http://research.flagler.edu:9017/stable/pdf/2678626.pdf.

Link, B.G., &Phelan, J.C.(2013). Labeling and stigma. In C.S. Aneshensel, J.C. Phelan, & A. Bierman, *Handbook of the sociology of mental health* (2nd ed.). New York: Springer.

Littlewood, R. (2002). *Pathologies of the west: An anthropology of mental illness in Europe and America.* New York: Cornell University Press.

Littrell, J. M. (1998). *Brief counseling in action.* New York: W.W. Norton and Company.

Livingston, J. D. (2013). Mental illness-related structural stigma: The downward spiral of systematic exclusion final report. *Calgary, Alberta:*

Mental Health Commission of Canada. Retrieved February 13, 2018 www.mentalhealthcommission.ca.

Lushin, V., & Anastas, J.W. (2011). Harm reduction in substance abuse treatment: Pragmatism as an epistemology for social work practice. *Journal of Social Work Practice 11*: 96-100. doi: 10.1080/1533256X.2011.546205.

MacDonald, P. (2016). 'The nowness of everything': A mindfulness-based approach to psychotherapy. *Psychodynamic practice 22*(1), 38-49 doi: 10.1080/14753634.2016.1126979

MacMaster, S. A. (2004). Harm reduction: A new perspective on substance abuse services. *Social Work 49* (3), 356-363. Retrieved from http://doctordeluca.com/Library/AbstinenceHR/HarmReductionNewPerspective04.pdf.

Malik, M. L. & Beutler, L. E. (2002). The emergence of dissatisfaction with the DSM. In M. L. Malik and L. E. Beutler (Eds.), *Rethinking the DSM: A Psychological Perspective* (3-15). Washington, DC: American Psychiatric Association.

Mander, G. (2000). *A psychodynamic approach to brief therapy.* London: Sage.

Maslow, A. (1943). Atheory of human motivation. *Psychological review 50*(4), 370-396.

Mead, H. (1934). *Mind, self, and society.* Chicago: University of Chicago Press.

Merriam-Webster. (2018). Madness. Retrieved from https://www.merriam-webster.com/dictionary/madness.

Miller, W. R., & Rollick, S. (2002). *Motivational interviewing: Preparing people for change* (2nd ed.). New York: Guilford Press.

Mills, C. W. (1959). *The sociological imagination.* New York: Oxford Press.

Mintz, S. (1995). *Moralists and modernizers: America's pre-civil war reformers.* Baltimore and London: The Johns Hopkins Press.

Minuchin, S., Lee, W., and Simon, G. (1996). *Mastering family therapy: Journeys of growth and transformation.* New York: John Wiley and Sons.

Mirowsky, J. and Ross, C.E. (1989). *Social causes of psychological distress.* Hawthorne, NY: Aldine de Gruyter.

National Association of Social Workers. (n.d.) www.socialworkers.org

National Alliance on Mental Illness (NAMI). (n.d.). ECT, TMS, and other brain stimulation therapies. Retrieved from https://www.nami.org/LearnMore/Treatment/ECT,-TMS-and-Other-Brain-Stimulation-Therapies.

National Center on Addiction and Substance Abuse at Columbia University. (2010). *Behind bars II: Substance abuse and America's prison population.* New York: Columbia University.

National Institute of Mental Health (NIMH). (2018). Intramural researchers develop suicide risk screening toolkit for medical settings. Retrieved from https://www.nimh.nih.gov/news/science-news/2018/intramural-researchers-develop-suicide-risk-screening-toolkit-for-medical-settings.shtml.

National Institute of Mental Health (NIMH). (n.d.) Any disorder among children. Retrieved from https://www.nimh.nih.gov/health/statistics/prevalence/any-disorder-among-children.shtml.

National Institute of Mental Health (NIMH). (n.d.) Any mental illness (AMI) among U.S. Adults. Retrieved from https://www.nimh.nih.gov/health/statistics/prevalence/any-mental-illness-ami-among-us-adults.shtml.

National Institution of Mental Health. (n.d.) Severe mental illness (SMI) among U.S. adults. Retrieved from https://www.nimh.nih.gov/health/statistics/prevalence/serious-mental-illness-smi-among-us-adults.shtml.

National Institute of Mental Health. (2016). Eating Disorders. Retrieved from https://www.nimh.nih.gov/health/topics/eating-disorders/index.shtml.

National Institute of Mental Health. (2016). Women and Mental Health. Retrieved https://www.nimh.nih.gov/health/topics/women-and-mental-health/index.shtml.

Newbigging, K., Ridley, J., McKeown, M., Sadd, J., Machin, K., Cruse, K., De La Haye, S., Able, L., & Poursanidou, K. (2015). *Independent mental health advocacy: The right to be heard.* London and Philadelphia: Jessica Kingsley Publishers.

Nichols, M. P., & Swartz, R. C. (2001). *Family therapy: Concepts and methods* (5th ed.). Boston: Allyn and Bacon.

Nolan, P., & Lenski, G. (2011). *Human societies: An introduction to macrosociology* (11th ed.). Boulder: Paradigm Publishers.

O'Brien, P.J. & Crowhurst, B. (2013). Pausing to consider the impact of cultural trends on mental health treatment. International Journal of Psychosocial Rehabilitation 17 (2), 105-118. Retrieved from http://www.psychosocial.com/IJPR_17/Pausing_to_consider_Cultural_Trends_O%27Brien.html.

Odar, C., Canter, K. S., & Roberts, M. C. (2013). Future directions for advancing issues in children's mental health: A Delphi cpoll. *Journal of Child and Family Studies* (22), 903-911 doi: 10.1007/s10826-012-9649-2

Oetzel, J., Duran, B., Yizhou, J., and Lucero, J. (2007). "Social support and undermining as correlates for alcohol, drug, and mental disorders in American Indian women presenting for primary care at an Indian Health Service hospital." *Journal of Health Communication.* 12. 187-206. Retrieved from http://research.flagler.edu:9839/eds/pdfviewer/pdfviewer?vid=1&sid=b8e6f55f-34f5-4c14-951c-2736b4b3c6db%40sessionmgr4010.

O'Hanlon, B. and Weiner-Davis, M. (1989). *In search of solutions: A new direction in psychotherapy.* New York: W.W. Norton and Company.

Olds, J. and Schwartz. (2009). *The lonely American: Drifting apart in the twenty-first century.* Boston: Beacon Press.

Olson, P. (1970). *The study of modern society: Perspectives from classic sociology.* New York: Random House.

Parsons, T. (1951). *The social system.* Glencoe, IL: The Free Press.

Pearson, G. (2013). DSM-5: What will it change? *Perspectives in Psychiatric Care, 49* (4), 219-220. doi: 10.1111/ppc.12041

Perry, J. W. (1974). *The far side of madness.* Englewood Cliffs, NJ: Prentice-Hall.

Phillips, D. C. (1970). Organicism in the late nineteenth and early twentieth centuries. *Journal of the History of Ideas 31*(3), 413-432.

Phillips, E. L. (1985). *A guide for therapists and patients to short-term psychotherapy.* Springhill, IL: Charles C. Thomas Publisher.

Pilgrim, D. (2014). Influencing mental health policy and planning: DSM–5 as a disciplinary challenge for psychology. *Review of General Psychology, 18*(4), 293-301. Retrieved from http://research.flagler.edu:9839/eds/pdfviewer/pdfviewer?vid=1&sid=c8de272a-2049-4d12-a67e-3d726ccfb196%40sessionmgr4007

Polgar, M. (2010). Mental health care in organizations and systems. In T. Scheid and T. Brown (Eds.), *A handbook for the study of mental health: Social contexts, theories, and systems* (2nd ed.), (pp. 499-509) Cambridge: Cambridge University Press.

Porter, R. (2002). *Madness: A brief history.* Oxford and New York: Oxford University Press.

Power, K. (2009). A public health model of mental health for the 21st century. In K. Thompson, J. A. Buck, and H. H. Goldman *Transforming mental health services: Implementing the federal agenda for change* (pp. 111-115). Arlington, VA: American Psychiatric Association.

Prochaska, J. O., & DiClemente, C. C. (1982). Transtheoretical therapy: Towards a more integrative model of change. *Psychotherapy, theory, research, and practice 19,* 276-288.

Ptakowski, K. K. (2012). Legislative advocacy: Putting your house in order. In S. L. Lustig, *Advocacy strategies for health and mental health strategies: From patients to policies* (pp. 51-63). New York: Springer Publishing Co.

Pugh, T., Hatzenbuehler, M., & Link, B. (2014). Structural stigma and mental illness. *National Academy of Science.* Retrieved from https://sites.nationalacademies.org/cs/groups/dbassesite/documents/webpage/dbasse_170045.pdf.

Rapaport, A. (1968). "Systems analysis: General systems theory," *International encyclopedia of the social sciences.* New York: Macmillan and Free Press. 15. P. 454.

Rasinski, K., Woll, P., and Cooke, A. (2005). Stigma and substance use disorders. In P.W. Corrigan (Ed.), *On the stigma of mental illness: Practical strategies for research and social change* (pp. 219-236). Washington: APA.

Ratts, M. J., Singh, A.A., Nassar-McMillan, S., Butler, S. K., & McCullough, J. R. (2016). Multicultural and social justice ounseling competencies: Guidelines for the counseling profession. *Journal of multicultural counseling and development, 44*(1), 28-48. doi: 10.1002/jmcd.12035

Ritzer, G. (2002). Introduction to McDonaldization. In *McDonaldization: The reader* (pp. 7-23). Thousand Oaks, London, and New Delhi: Pine Forge Press.

Robbins, S. P. (2014). From the Editor—The DSM-5 and its role in social work assessment and research. *Journal of Social Work Education, 50,* 201-205. doi: 10.1080/10437797.2014.885363

Roberts, J. L., & Weeks, E. (2007). Stigmatizing the unhealthy. *Journal of Law, Medicine and Ethics, 45,* 484-491. Retrieved from http://research.flagler.edu:9839/eds/pdfviewer/pdfviewer?vid=1&sid=2f3a611f-50d7-416f-aba9- 5c2b97591bd7%40sessionmgr4007.

Rogers, C. (1970). *Carl Rogers on encounter groups.* New York, Evanston, and London: Harper and Row.

Rosen, G. (1968). *Madness in society: Chapters in the historical sociology of mental illness.* New York: Harper Touchbook.

Rosenhan, D. L. (1973). On being sane in insane places. *Science 179*(4070), 250-258 Retrieved from http://research.flagler.edu:9017/stable/pdf/1735662.pdf.

Royster, M. (2012). The success and failure of scared straight: A reassessment of juvenile delinquency deterrent methods and their measurements. *The International Journal of Interdisciplinary Social Sciences 6* (8), 145-151. Retrieved from http://research.flagler.edu:9838/eds/pdfviewer/pdfviewer?vid=1&sid=11c7fa24-285c-461f-90fe-d95cbcd991f4%40sessionmgr102

Salerno, R. A. (2004). *Beyond the enlightenment: Lives and thoughts of social theorists.* Westport, CN: Praeger.

Sandstrom, K. L., Lively, K. J., Martin, D. D., & Fine, G. A. (2014). *Symbols, selves and social reality: A symbolic interactionist approach to social psychology and sociology* (4th ed.). New York: Oxford University Press.

Sayegh, C. S., Huey, S. J. Jr., Zara, E. J., & Jhaveri, K. (2017). Follow-up treatment effects of continency management on substance abuse: A meta-analysis. *Psychology of addictive behaviors 31*(1), 403-414. doi: 10.1037/adb0000277

Scarf, M. (1980). *Unfinished business: Pressure points in the lives of women.* New York: Ballantine Books.

Scheff, T. (1999). *Being mentally ill: A sociological theory* (3rd ed.). New York: Aldine de Gruyter.

Scheid, T. L. (2004). *Tie and knot and hang on: Providing mental health care in a turbulent environment.* New York: Aldine de Gruyter.

Scheid, T., & Brown, T. (2010). Mental health systems and policy (2nd ed.). In T. Scheid and T.

Brown (Eds.), *A handbook for the study of mental health: Social contexts, theories, and systems* (407-419). Cambridge: Cambridge University Press.

Scott, C. H. (1976). *Lester Frank Ward.* Boston: Twayne Publishers.

Scott, S., & Thorpe, C. (2006). The sociological imagination of R.D. Laing. *Sociological theory 24*(4), 331-352.

Scull, A. T. (1977). *Decarceration: Community treatment and the deviant—A radical view.* Englewood Cliffs, NJ: Prentice-Hall.

Scull, A.W. (2009). *Hysteria: The biography.*Oxford, UK: Oxford University Press.

Scull, A. (2015). *Madness in civilization: A cultural history of insanity from the Bible to Freud, from the madhouse to modern medicine.* Princeton and Oxford: Oxford University Press.

Shaffer, J. B.P., & Galinsky, D. (1989). *Models of group therapy.* Engelwood Cliffs, NJ: Prentice Hall.

Sherman, C. (2001). *How to go to therapy: Making the most of professional help.* New York: Atrandom.com.

Shireman, J. F. (2015). *Critical issues in child welfare.* New York: Columbia University Press. Shorter, E. (1992). *From paralysis to fatigue: A history of psychosomatic illness in the modern era.* New York: Free Press.

Shorter, E. (2015). *What psychiatry left out of the DSM-5: Historical mental disorders today.* New York and London: Routledge.

Singer, M., & Page, J. B. (2014). *The social value of drug addicts: Uses of the useless.* Walnut Creek, CA: Left Coast Press.

Singh, R. D., Jimerson, S. R., Renshaw, T., Saeki, E., Hart, S. R., Earhart, J., & Stewart, K. (2011). A summary and synthesis of contemporary empirical evidence regarding the effects of the drug abuse resistance education program (D.A.R.E.). *Contemporary School Psychology 15*, 93-102. Retrieved from https://research.flagler.edu:11243/fulltext/EJ934709.pdf

Smith, S. R., & Hamon, R. R. (2012). *Exploring family theories* (3rd ed.). New York and Oxford: Oxford University Press.

Sorokin, Pitirim A. (1941). *The crisis of our age.* New York: E.P. Dutton and Co.

Spitz, H. I., & Spitz, S. T. (1999). *A pragmatic approach to group psychotherapy.* Philadelphia and London: Brunner/Mazel.

Spitzer, R. L. (1975). On pseudoscience and science, logic in remission, any psychiatric diagnosis: A critique of Rosenhan's on being sane in insane places. *Journal of abnormal psychology 84*(5), 442-452. Retrieved from http://research.flagler.edu:9838/eds/pdfviewer/pdfviewer?vid=1&sid=dd56d575-bc12-4844-b10a-26e10a8b938b%40sessionmgr103.

Stewart, N. R., Winborn, B. B., Burks, H. M. Jr., Johnson, R.C., & Engelkes, J. E. (1978). *Systematic counseling.* Englewood Cliffs, NJ: Prentice-Hall, Inc.

Substance Abuse Mental Health and Services Administration. (2015). Results from the 2015 national survey on drug use and health: Detailed tables. Retrieved from https://www.samhsa.gov/data/sites/default/files/NSDUH-DetTabs-2015/NSDUH-DetTabs-2015/NSDUH-DetTabs-2015.htm.

Sugie, N. F., & Turney, K. (2017). Beyond incarceration: Criminal justice contact and mental health. *American Sociological Review 82*(4), 714-743. doi: 10.1177/0003122417713188

Sullivan, H. S. (1953). *The interpersonal theory of psychiatry.* New York: W.W. Norton and Company.

Szasz, T. (1961). *The myth of mental illness: Foundations of a theory of personal conduct.* New York: Harper.

Talbott, J. A. (1978). *The death of the asylum: A critical study of state hospital management, services and care.* New York: Grune & Stratton.

Tatarsky, A. & Marlatt, G. A. (2010). State of the art in harm reduction psychotherapy: An emerging treatment for substance misuse. *Journal of Clinical Psychology, 66* (2), 117-122. doi: 10.1002/jclp.20672

Thomas, W.I., & Thomas, D. S. (1928). *The child in America: Behavior problems and programs.* New York: Knopf.

Thomas, A. R. (1998). Ronald Reagan and the commitment of the mentally ill: Capital, interest groups and the eclipse of social policy. *Electronic Journal of Sociology.* Retrieved from http://www.sociology.org/ejs-archives/vol003.004/thomas.html.

Timascheff, N. S. (1967). *Sociological theory: Its nature and growth* (4th ed.). New York: Random House.

Tocqueville, A. (1835 & 1840/2000). *Democracy in America,* H. Reeve (Trans.). New York: Bantam.

Torrey, E. F. (1997). *Out of the shadows: Confronting America's mental illness crisis.* New York: John Wiley and Sons.

Torrey, E. F., & Miller, J. (2001). *The invisible plague: The rise of mental illness from 1750 to the present.* New Brunswick, NJ and London: Rutgers University Press.

Totten, N. (2003). *Body psychotherapy: An introduction.* Berkshire, UK: Open University Press.

Tuckman, B. (1965). Developmental sequences in small groups. *Psychological Bulletin.* 63 (6), 384-399.

Turkel, S. (2011). *Alone together: Why we expect more from technology and less from each other.* New York: Basic Books.

Turney-High, H. H. (1968). *Man and system: Foundations for the study of human relations.* New York: Appleton-Century-Crofts.

Velez-Agosto, N. M., Soto-Crespo, J. G., Vizcarrondo-Oppenheim, M., Vega-Molina, S., & Garcia, C. (2017). Bronfenbrenner's bioecological theory revision: Moving culture from the macro into the micro. *Perspectives on psychological science 12*(5), 900-910. doi: 10.1177/1745691617704397

Vestal, C. (2017). Meth use surges in western, southern, and midwestern states. *Governing the States.* Retrieved from http://www.governing.com/topics/public-justice-safety/sl-meth-usage-drugs-states-illegal.html.

Wakefield, J. C. (2013). DSM-5 and clinical social work: Mental disorder and psychological justice as goals of clinical intervention. *Clinical Social Work Journal, 41,* 131–138. Retrieved from http://research.flagler.edu:9838/eds/pdfviewer/pdfviewer?vid=1&sid=f4cbacff-8130-485b-9117-704172b3f0be%40sessionmgr120.

Walther, W. A., Abelson, S., & Malmon, A. (2014). Active minds: Creating peer-to-peer mental health awareness. *Journal of college student psychotherapy 28*(1), 12-22. doi: 10.1080/87568225.2014.854673

Watson, D. P. (2012). The evolving understanding of recovery: What does the sociology of mental health have to offer? *Humanity & Society* 36(4), 290-308. doi: 10.1177/0160597612458904.

Watters, E. (2011). *Crazy like us: The globalization of the American psyche.* New York: Free Press.

Weber, M. (1905/2003). *The Protestant Ethic and the Spirit of Capitalism.* Trans. By Talcott Parsons with a foreword by R.H. Tawney. Mineola, NY: Dover Publications, Inc.

Weiner, B. (1975). On being sane in insane places: A process (attributional) analysis and critique. *Journal of abnormal psychology 84*(5), 433-441. Retrieved from http://research.flagler.edu:9838/eds/detail/detail?vid=0&sid=9ab3fffd-4cf2-4016-bce0-542af2d46f69%40sessionmgr101&bdata=JnNpdGU9ZWRzLWxpdmUmc2NvcGU9c2l0ZQ%3d%3d#AN=1975-32013-001&db=pdh.

Whitaker, R. (2002). *Mad in America: Bad science, bad medicine, and the enduring mistreatment of the mentally ill.* New York: Basic Books.

Whitaker, R. (2015). *Anatomy of an epidemic: Magic bullets, psychiatric drugs and the astonishing rise of mental illness in America.* New York: Broadway Books.

White, W. (2014). *Slaying the dragon: The history of addiction treatment and recovery in America* (2nd ed.) Bloomington, IL: Chestnut Health Systems/Lighthouse Institute.

Wilks, T. (2012). *Advocacy for social work practice.* Berkshire, UK: Open University Press.

Winbolt, B. (2011). *Solution-focused therapy for the helping professions.* London and Philadelphia: Jessica Kingsley Publishers.

World Health Organization. (2003). Advocacy for mental health: Mental health policy and service guidance package. Retrieved from http://www.who.int/mental_health/resources/en/Advocacy.pdf

World Health Organization. (2016). Mental health: Strengthening our response. Retrieved from www.who.int/news-room/fact-sheets/detail/mental-health-strengthening-our-response

Yalom, I. D. (1989). *Love's executioner and other tales of psychotherapy.* New York: HarperPerennial.

Zalaquett, C. P., Fuerth, K. M., Stein, C., Ivey, A. E., & Bradford Ivey, M. (2008). Reframing the DSM-IV-TR from a multicultural/social justice perspective. *Journal of Counseling and Development Summer, 86,* 364-371. Retrieved from http://research.flagler.edu:9838/eds/pdfviewer/pdfviewer?vid=1&sid=4aee64c7-b8b2-4977-b7c2-608bd8dc3535%40sessionmgr104.

Zwelling, S. S. (1985). *Quest for a cure: The public hospital in Williamsburg, Virginia, 1773-1885.* Williamsburg, VA: The Colonial Williamsburg Foundation.

INDEX

T

W

www.ingramcontent.com/pod-product-compliance
Ingram Content Group UK Ltd.
Pitfield, Milton Keynes, MK11 3LW, UK
UKHW020800290926
15470UKWH00008B/1832/J

9 781622 7332